Physical Pharmaceutics - I
Revised Edition

Physical Pharmaceutics – I
Revised Edition

Dr. Suryadevara Vidyadhara

Principal, Chebrolu Hanumaiah Institute of Pharmaceutical Sciences,
(Formerly N.E.S. Institute of Pharmaceutical Sciences),
Chandramoulipuram, Chowdavaram, Guntur-19. A.P.

Dr. Ramesh Babu.Janga

Prof in Pharmaceutics
Chebrolu Hanumaiah Institute of Pharmaceutical Sciences,
Guntur.

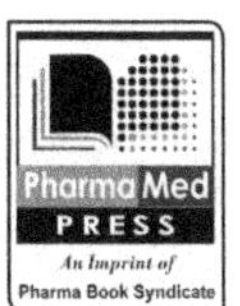

PharmaMed Press

An imprint of Pharma Book Syndicate

A Unit of BSP Books Pvt. Ltd.
4-4-309/316, Giriraj Lane,
Sultan Bazar, Hyderabad - 500 095.

Physical Pharmaceutics-I, Revised Edition *by Suryadevara Vidyadhara and Janga Ramesh Babu*

© 2016, by Publisher

Published by

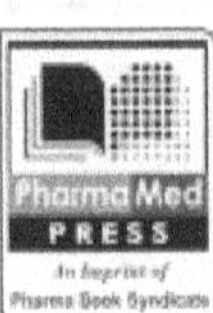

PharmaMed Press

An imprint of Pharma Book Syndicate

A unit of BSP Books Pvt. Ltd.
4-4-309/316, Giriraj Lane, Sultan Bazar, Hyderabad - 500 095.
Phone: 040-23445605, 23445688; Fax: 91+40-23445611
e-mail: info@pharmamedpress.com

ISBN : 978-93-5230-115-7 (HB)

Preface

The authors are pleased to bring out the Second edition of Physical Pharmaceutics I. This book is written specially to provide the coverage of syllabus for students of Under Graduate, Post Graduate and some areas of Research Level in the subject of Pharmaceutical Formulations as Physical Pharmacy. The subject of Physical Pharmacy has been associated with Physico chemical properties of substances and gives an idea about Theoretical Principles which can be applied in the Development Of Formulations of any Dosage Forms.

This book contains 08 chapters which covers the syllabus of most of the Indian Universities. The salient features of this book in the presentation of fundamental concepts in a very simplified and self explanatory form. It is expected that present text book of Physical Pharmaceutics- I would facilitate in laying a sound foundation in students for Pharmaceutics. We have considered various comments made by different readers and tried to avoid those comments and make it accurate in this issue.

We are grateful to the management of Nagarjuna Education Society (NES) and Chebrolu Hanumaiah Institute of Pharmaceutical Sciences (CHIPS), Guntur, for constant encouragement provided during completion of this Book.

The authors would like to thank to all the Faculty Members and Students of CHIPS, Friends and Family Members who have been the source of Inspiration in the preparation of this Book.

We are sincerely extend out thanks to Pharma Med Press for kind Co-operation and immense interest taken in bringing out this book.

The Authors have made every attempt, strived hand to present a nice and good book. We would appreciate any suggestions and comments from Students, Fellow Teachers and Research Scholars for future improvement of this Book.

- Authors

Contents

Chapter 1

States of Matter

Chapter 2
Thermodynamics

Chapter 3
Physical Properties of Drug Molecules

Chapter 4
Solutions of Non-electrolytes

Chapter 5
Solutions of Electrolytes

Chapter 6
Ionic Equilibria

Chapter 7
Buffers and Buffered Isotonic Solutions

Chapter 8

Electrochemistry

Chapter 9

Viscosity

Chapter 10
Photochemistry

STATES OF MATTER

1.1 Introduction

Matter exists in three different physical forms. They are namely – gases, liquids and solids.

The molecules of the solids are held very close to each other. And the solids became of their close proximity between the molecules generally exits as compact masses. In the liquids, the arrangement of the molecules is not so compact when compared to solids. Hence the liquids take the shape of a container. In gases the molecules are very spaciously placed. They are very far from each other. The inter conversion of these three physical forms – solid-liquid-gases is possible (in a specified way and vice versa generally). But when we consider the solids with high vapour pressure, they directly convert into the gaseous state without passing through the liquid state. This process is called as sublimation, and the reconversion is known as deposition.

Sometimes the matter can also exist in another phase (4th phase) mesophase. It is also called liquid crystalline state which is an intermediate state between the liquids and crystalline solids.

1.2 Binding Forces Among the Molecules

Generally for the matter to exist in the form of liquid or solid or gas an association must exist between the molecules. The binding forces between the molecules are of different types.

Repulsive forces: When the molecules are brought so close that the outer charge causes them to repel each other like rigid elastic bodies.

The repulsion is due to the interpenetration of the electronic clouds of molecules and increases exponentially with a decrease in distance between the molecules. At certain equilibrium distance about (3 to 4) $\times$ 10^{-8} cm (3-4A°) the repulsive and attractive forces are equal.

Attractive forces: Generally when two atoms or molecules are brought closer together, the opposite charges and binding forces in the two molecules are closer together than the similar charges and forces causing the molecules to attract one another.

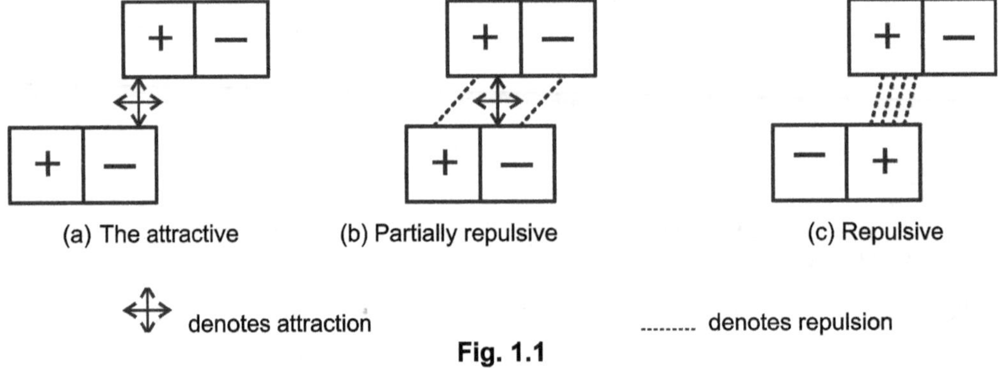

Fig. 1.1

Vander Waals forces: Generally the dipolar molecules tend to align themselves to form a group which became an attraction between the two opposite poles of the molecules. The South Pole is attracted towards the North Pole and vice-versa. These dipole-dipole interactions are called as keesom forces.

The dipoles are able to polarise a non polar molecule and there after aligns with them and that type of interactions are called dipole-induced dipole or debye interactions.

The nonpolar molecules are able to induce the polarity to each other there by resulting in induced-dipole-induced dipole interactions also called as London attractions.

The Vander Waals forces are applicable in the process of condensation of gases.

- Solubility of drugs
- Formation of some metal complexes and molecular addition compounds
- Some biological processes and drug actions

Generally the intermolecular forces like London forces, Keesom forces and Debye interactions are referred as Vander Waal's forces. But generally the London forces alone are referred as Vander Waal's forces because they are the interactions between the non-polar molecules.

Ion Dipole and Ion-induced Dipole Forces: These types of forces between the molecules are specially concerned with the parameter of solubility. And these interactions increase the solubility of substances.

Hydrogen Bonding: The bonding that exists between a molecule containing the hydrogen atom and strong electro-negative atoms is referred to as hydrogen bonding.

Hydrogen bonding is of two types.

Intermolecular Hydrogen Bonding: The hydrogen bond which is formed between two molecules is referred to as intermolecular hydrogen bonding.

e.g.,   Hydrogen fluoride   Formic acid dimmer (CHOOH)

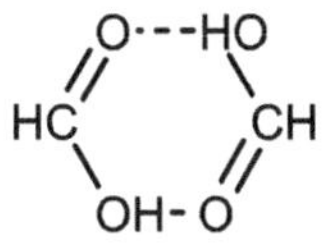

F-H---F-H

$\rightarrow$ Hydrogen bond

Intramolecular Hydrogen Bonding: The hydrogen bond which is formed between two atoms of the same molecule is referred to as intramolecular hydrogen bonding.

e.g.,   Salicylic acid

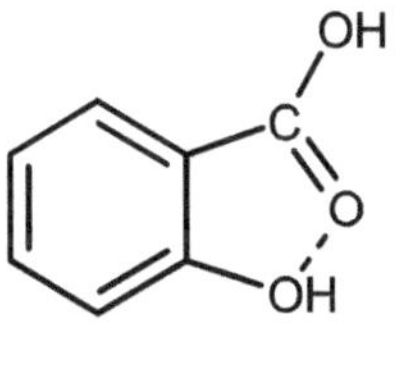

Bond Type	Bond energy (kcal/mole (appron))
Vander Waals force and other inter molecules attraction	
Dipole-Dipole interactions, orientation effect or keesom force	
Dipole-induced dipole interactions, induction effect, Debye force	1-10
Induced dipole-induced dipole interaction, dispersion effect or London force	

Ion dipole interactions

Hydrogen bonds   O-H---O $\rightarrow$ 6   C-H---O $\rightarrow$ 2-3

                      O-H---N $\rightarrow$ 4-7   N-H---O$\rightarrow$2-3   F-H---F$\rightarrow$7

The Gaseous State: Gases have neither definite shape nor definite volume as the molecules in this state are far apart from one another. They occupy the entire volume of any given container and their volume is assumed to be the same as that of the container. As the gas molecules travel in random paths, frequently colliding with one another and with the walls of the container in which they are confined, they exert a pressure.

The Ideal Gas Law: A gas which obeys all the gas laws under all the conditions of temperature and pressure is called ideal gas. The gases which do not obey gas laws under required conditions are called real gases. Real gases show the behaviour of ideal gas at high temperatures and low pressures.

The ideal gas equation is obtained by combining the three gas laws. They are Boyles law, Charles law and Avagadro's law.

Boyles Law: It is defined as the volume of a given mass of a gas is inversely proportional to pressure at constant temperature

$$V \alpha \frac{1}{P} \quad (or) \quad P \alpha \frac{1}{V}$$

$$PV = k \text{ (constant)} \quad\quad\quad\quad .....(1.1)$$

Charles-Gay Lussac Law: At constant pressure, the volume of a given mass of a gas at 0 °C increases or decreases by 1/273 times its volume for every degree rise or fall in temperature i.e., the volume of a gas increased linearly with increase of temperature if pressure is constant

$$V \propto T$$

$$V = kT \quad\quad\quad\quad .....(1.2)$$

Both eq. (1.1) and (1.2) are combined to obtain the relationship

$$\frac{PV}{T} = k \text{ (constant)} \quad\quad\quad\quad .....(1.3)$$

The constant k depends upon the amount of the gas. We can understand from Avagadro's law.

Avagadro's Law: It states that equal volumes of all gases, measured under the same conditions of temperature and pressure, contain equal number of molecules. A mole of a substance contains a fixed no of molecules, applying this law it can be concluded that equal volumes of all gases, measured under the same conditions of temperature and pressure, contain equal number of moles. Then we have

$$k \propto n \quad \text{or} \quad k = nR$$

where 'R' is called molar gas constant and independent of the amount of gas taken

$$\frac{PV}{T} = nR$$

$$\boxed{PV = nRT}$$

The value of gas constant 'R' is same for all gases, hence it is called universal gas constant. To obtain numeric value for R, let us proceed as follows: If 1 mole of an ideal gas is chosen, its volume under standard conditions of temperature and pressure (STP) (i.e., at 0 °C and 760 mm Hg) has been found to be 22.414 lit.

$$1 \text{ atm} \times 22.414 \text{ lit} = 1 \text{ mole} \times R \times 273.16 \text{ °K}$$

$$R = 0.08205 \text{ lit atm/mole deg}$$

The molar gas constant may also be given in energy units by expressing the pressure in dyne/cm^2 (1 atm = 1.0133 × 10^6, volume in cm^3 is 22,414 cm^3). Then

$$R = \frac{PV}{T} = \frac{\left(1.0133 \times 10^6\right) \times 22,414}{273.16°}$$

$$= 8.314 \times 10^7 \text{ erg/mole deg}$$

or since 1 joule = 10^7 erg

$$R = 8.314 \text{ Joules/mole deg}$$

The constant can also be expressed in cal/mole deg employing the equivalent, 1 cal = 4.184 joules.

$$R = \frac{8.314 \text{ joules/(mole deg)}}{4.184 \text{ joules/cal}} = 1.987 \text{ cal/ mole deg}$$

Molecular Weight: The approximate molecular weight of a gas can be determined by use of ideal gas law. The number of moles of gas n is replaced by its equivalent g/M in which g is the grams of gas and M is molecular weight.

$$PV = g/M \, (RT)$$

$$M = \frac{gRT}{PV}$$

Kinetic Molecular Theory: The equations just given have been formulated from experimental consideration. This theory was developed to explain the behaviour of gases and to lend additional support to the rancidity of the gas laws is called the kinetic molecular theory. Some of the more important statements of the theory are the following

1. Gases are composed of particles called molecules, the total volume of which is so small as to be negligible in relation to the volume of the space in which the molecules are confined. This condition is approximated in actual gases only at low pressures and high temperatures in which case the molecules of the gas are far apart.

2. The particles of the gas do not attract one another but rather move with complete independence, again this statement applies only at low pressures.

3. The particles exhibit continuous random motion owing to their kinetic energy. The average kinetic energy, E, is directly proportional to the absolute temperature of the gas or

$$E = \frac{3}{2}RT$$

4. The molecules exhibit perfect elasticity, that is there is no net loss of speed after they collide with one another and with the walls of the confining vessel which latter effect accounts for the gas pressure. Although the net velocity and therefore the average kinetic energy, does not change on collision, the speed and energy of the individual molecules may differ widely at any instant.

From these and other postulates, the following fundamental kinetic equation is derived:

$$PV = \frac{1}{3}nmc^2$$

where P is the pressure and V the volume occupied by any number n of molecules of mass m having an average velocity $\bar{c}$.

Using the fundamental equation, the root mean square velocity $\left(c^2\right)^{\frac{1}{2}}$ (usually written μ) of the molecules is an ideal gas can be obtained. Solving for c^2 in $M = \left(\dfrac{gRT}{PV}\right)$ and taking the square root of both sides of the equation leads to the formula.

$$\mu = \sqrt{\frac{3PV}{nm}} = \sqrt{\frac{3RT}{M}} = \sqrt{\frac{3P}{d}}$$

Since the term nm/V is equal to density

In other words, the rate of diffusion of a gas is inversely proportional to the square root of its density. Such a relation confirms the early findings of Graham, who showed that a light gas diffused more rapidly through a porous membrane than diffued a heavier one.

Vander Waals Equation for Real Gases: The fundamental kinetic equation is found to compare with the ideal gas equation, since the kinetic theory is based on the assumption of the ideal state. However, real gases are not composed of infinitely small and perfectly elastic non attracting spheres. Instead, they are composed of molecules of a finite volume that tend to attract one another. These factors affect the volume and pressure term in the ideal equation, so that certain refinements must be incorporated if ideal gas equation is to provide results that check with experiment. A number of such expressions have been suggested, the Vander Waals equation being one of the best known of there for 1 mole of gas, the Vander Waals equation is written as

$$\left(P + \frac{a}{V^2} \right)(V - b) = RT$$

for n moles of gas in container of volume V is

$$\left(P + \frac{an^2}{V^2} \right)(V - nb) = nRT$$

The term a/V^2 accounts for the internal pressure per mole resulting from intermolecular forces of attraction between the molecules b accounts for the incompressibility of the molecules, that is excluded volume, which is about four times the molecular volume. Polar liquids have high internal pressure and serve as solvents only for substances of similar internal pressure. Non polar molecules have low internal pressure and are not able to overcome the powerful cohesive forces of the polar solvent molecules. Mineral oil is immiscible with water for this reason. When the volume of a gas is large, a/V^2 and b becomes insignificant with respect to P and V, respectively. Under these conditions the Vander Waals' equation for 1 mole of gas reduces to ideal gas equation, PV = RT, and of low pressures, real gases behave in an ideal manner.

1.3 The Liquid State

Liquefication of Gases: When a gas is cooled, it loses some of its kinetic energy in the form of heat, and the velocity of the molecules decreases. If pressure is applied to the gas, the molecules are brought within the sphere of the Vander Waals interaction forces and pass into liquid state. Because of these forces, liquids are considerably denser than gases and occupy a definite volume. The transitions from a gas to a liquid and from a liquid to solid depend not only on the temperature, but also on the pressure to which the substance is subjected.

If the temperature is elevated sufficiently, a value is reached above which it is impossible to liquefy a gas, irrespective of the pressure applied. This temperature above which a liquid can no longer exist is known as the critical temperature. The pressure required to liquefy a gas at its critical temperature is the critical pressure, which is also the highest vapour pressure that the liquid can have. The farther a gas is cooled below its critical temperature the less pressure is required to liquefy it. Based on this principle, all known gases have been liquefied.

The critical temperature of water is 374 ^{0}C or 647 ^{0}K and its critical pressure is 218 atm, while the corresponding values for helium are 5.2 $^{\circ}$K and 2.26 atm. The critical temperature serves as a rough measure of the attractive forces between molecules, for at temperatures above the critical value, the molecules posses sufficient kinetic energy so that no amount of pressure can bring them within the range of attractive forces that cause the particles to stick together. The high critical values for water result because of the strong dipolar forces between the molecules and particularly the hydrogen bonding that exits. Conversely helium molecules are attracted only by the weak London force and consequently this element must be cooled to the extremely low temperature of 5.2 $^{\circ}$K before it can be liquefied. Above this critical temperature, helium remains as a gas no matter what the pressure.

Method of Achieving Liquefication: One of the most obvious ways to liquefy a gas is to subject it to intense cold by the use of freezing mixture. Other methods depend on the cooling effect produced in a gas as it expands. Thus, suppose we allow an ideal gas to expand so rapidly that no heat enter the system, such an expansion is termed as adiabatic expansion, may be achieved by carrying out the process in a Dewar, (or) Vacuum flask which effectively insulates the contents of the flask from the external environment. The work that has to be done to bring about expansion therefore must come from the gas itself at the expense of its own heat energy content. As a result, the temperature of the gas falls. If this procedure is repeated a sufficient number of times, the total drop in temperature may be sufficient to cause liquefication of the gas.

A cooling effect is also observed when a highly compressed non ideal gas expands, into a region of low pressure. In this case the drop in temperature results from the energy expanded in over coming the cohesive forces of attraction between the molecules. This cooling effect is known as Joule-Thomson effect and differs from the cooling produced in adiabatic expansion, in which the gas does external work. To bring about liqueficatin by the Joule Thomson effect, it may be necessary to precool the gas before allowing it to expand. Liquid oxygen and liquid air are obtained by methods based on this effect.

Aerosols: Gases can be liquefied under high pressure, provided if it is at below the critical temperature. When the pressure is reduced, the molecules expand and the liquid reverts to a gas. This reversible change of state is the basic principle involved in the preparation of pharmaceutical aerosols. In such products a drug is dissolved or suspended in a propellant, a material that is liquid under the pressure conditions existing inside the container but forms a gas under normal atmospheric conditions. The container is so designed that, by depressing a volume, some of the drug propellant mixture is expelled owing to the excess pressure inside the container. If the drug is non-volatile it forms a fine spray as it leaves the valve orifice at the sometime, the liquid propellant vapourises off. The propellant used in these products is frequently a mixture of fluorinated hydrocarbons, although other gases, such as nitrogen and CO_2 are increasingly used. By varying the proportions of the various propellent it is possible to produce pressures within the container ranging from 1 to 6 atm at room temperature. Alternate fluorocarbon propellants that do not deplete the ozone layer of the atmosphere are perfectly used for investigation.

The containers are filled either by cooling the propellant and drug to a low temperature within the container, which is then sealed with the valve, or by sealing the drug in the container at room temperature and then forcing the required amount of propellant into the container under pressure. In both cases, when the product is at room temperature, part of the propellant is in the gaseous state and exerts the pressure necessary to extrude the drug, while the remainder is in liquid state and provides a solution or suspension vehicle for the drug.

The formulation of pharmaceuticals as aerosols is continuously increasing, since the method frequently offers distinct advantages over some of the more conventional methods of formulation. Thus antiseptic materials can be sprayed on to abraded skin with the minimum of discomfort to the patient. More significant is the increased efficiency often observed and the facility with which medication can be introduced into body cavities and passages.

Vapour Pressure of Liquids: Translational energy of motion (kinetic energy) is not distributed evenly among molecules, some of the molecules have more energy and hence higher velocities than others at any moment when a liquid is placed in an evacuated container at a constant temperature, the molecules with the highest energies break away from the surface of the liquid and pass into the gaseous state, and some of the molecules subsequently return to the liquid state, or condense when the rate of condensation equals the rate of vapourisation at a definite temperature, the vapour becomes saturated and a dynamic equilibrium is established. The pressure of the saturated vapour above the liquid is then known as the equilibrium vapour pressure. If a manometer is fitted to an evacuated vessel containing the liquid it is possible to obtain a record of the vapour pressure in millimetre of mercury. The pressure of a gas such as air, above the liquid would decrease the rate of evaporation, but it would not effect the equilibrium pressure of the vapour.

As the temperature of the liquid is evaluated more molecules approach the velocity necessary for escape and pass into gaseous state. As a result the vapour pressure increases with rising temperature as shown in Fig.1.2. At any point on one of the curves represents a condition in which the liquid and the vapour exist together in equilibrium. As observed in Fig. 1.2 if the temperature of any of the liquids is increased while the pressure is held constant or if the pressure is decreased while the temperature is held constant all the liquid will pass into vapour state.

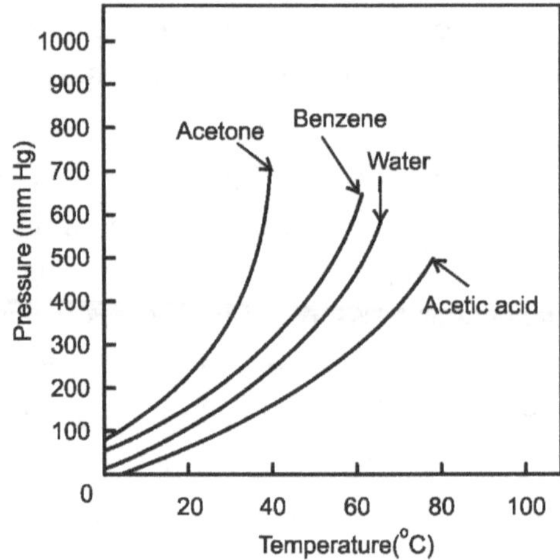

Fig. 1.2 The variation of the vapour pressure of some liquids with temperature

Clausius Calpeyron Equation: The relationship between the vapour pressure and the absolute temperature of liquids expressed by Clausius-Clapeyron equation.

$$\log \frac{P_2}{P_1} = \frac{\Delta Hv (T_2 - T_1)}{2.303\ RT_1T_2}$$

where P_1, P_2 are the vapour pressure at absolute temperature T_1, T_2, ΔHv is molar heat of vapourisation i.e., the heat absorbed by 1 mole of liquid when it passes into vapour state.

Boiling Point: If a liquid is placed in an open container and heated until the vapour pressure equals the atmospheric pressure, the vapour is seen to form bubbles that rise rapidly through the liquid and escape into gaseous state. The temperature at which the vapour pressure of the liquid equals to the external or atmospheric pressure is known as boiling point. All the absorbed heat is used to change the liquid to vapour, and the temperature dose not rise until the liquid is completely vapourised. At high elevation, the atmospheric pressure decreases and boiling point is lowered. At pressure of 700 mmHg, water boils at 97.7 °C at 17.5 mmHg it boils at 20 °C.

The heat that is absorbed when water vaporises at the normal boiling point is 539 cal/gm or about 9720 cal/mole for benzene if its 91.4 cal/gm at normal boiling point of 80.2 °C. These quantities of heat is known as latent heat of vaporisation. The boiling point may be considered as temperature at which thermal agitation can overcome the attractive forces between the molecules of a liquid. Therefore the boiling point of a compound, like the heat of vapourisation and the vapour pressure at a definite temperature, provides a rough indication of the magnitude of attractive forces.

The boiling point of normal hydrocarbons, simple alcohols and carboxylic acids increase with molecular weight, since the attractive Vander Waals forces become greater, with increasing number of atom branching of the chain produces a less compact molecule with reduced intermolecular attraction, and a decrease in the boiling point results. In general, the alcohol boils at a much higher temperature than saturated hydrocarbons of the same molecular weight because of association of alcohol through hydrogen bonding that can remain even in vapour state, the boiling of straight chain primary alcohols and carboxylic acid increase about 18 °C for each additional methylene group. Non polar substances, the molecules of which are held together by London forces, have low boiling point. Polar molecules particularly those such as ethylalcohol and water which are attracted through hydrogen bonding exhibit high boiling point.

1.4 Solids and Crystalline State

Crystalline Solids: The structural units of crystalline solids such as ice, sodium chloride and menthol are arranged in fixed geometric pattern or lattices. Crystalline solids, unlike liquids and gases have definite shapes and an orderly arrangement of units. Gases are easily compressed whereas solids, like liquids are practically incompressible. Crystalline solids show definite melting points, passing rather sharply from the solid to the liquid state. The various crystal forms are divided into six distinct crystal systems. They are together with examples of each cubic (NaCl), tetragonal (urea) hexagonal (Iodoform) rhombic iodine, monoclinic (sucrose), and triclinic (boric acid).

The units that constitute the crystal structure can be atom, molecules or ions. The sodium chloride crystal consists of cubic lattice of sodium ions interpenetrated by a lattice of chloride ions, the binding force of crystal being the electrostatic attraction of the oppositely charged ions. In diamond and graphite, the lattice units consists of atom held together by covalent bonds. Solid carbon dioxide, hydrogen chloride, and naphthalene form crystals composed of molecules as the binding units. In organic compounds the molecules are held together by Vander Waals forces and hydrogen bonding, which account for the weak binding and for low melting points of these crystals. Aliphatic hydrocarbon crystallize with their chain lying in a parallel arrangement, while fatty acids crystallize in layers of dimers with the chain lying parallel or tilted at an angle with respect to the base plane. Whereas ionic and atomic crystals in general are hard and brittle and have high melting points, molecular crystals are soft and have low melting points.

Metallic crystals are composed of positively charged ions in a field of freely moving electrons, sometimes called the electron gas. Metals are good conductors of electricity because of the free movement of the electrons in the lattice. Metals may be soft or hard or soft and have low or high melting points. The hardness and strength of metals depend in part on the kind of imperfection, or lattice defects in the crystals.

X-Ray Diffraction: X-rays are diffracted by crystals just as visible light is dispersed in a colour spectrum by a rule grating (i.e., a piece of glass with fine parallel lines of equal with drawn on it). This is due to the fact that x-rays have wavelengths of about the same magnitude as the distance between the atoms or molecules of crystals. The x-ray diffractions pattern is photographed on a sensitive plate arranged behind the crystals and by such a method the structure of a crystal may be investigated. Employing a later modification of this principle, involving reflection of the x-ray beam from the atomic planes of the crystals it has become possible to determine the distances of the various planes of crystal lattice. The structure of various compounds can be determined in this way.

Where whole crystals are unavailable or unsuitable for analysis, a powder of the substance may be investigated, comparing the position and intensity of the lines on such a diagram with corresponding lines on the photographs of as known sample allows one to conduct a qualitative and a quantitative chemical analysis.

The electron density and accordingly, the position of the atoms in complex structures such as pencillin may be determined from a mathematical study of the data obtained by x-ray diffraction.

Melting Point and Heat of Fusion: The temperature at which a liquid passes into the solid state is known as the freezing point. It is also the melting point or melting point of a pure crystalline solid is strictly defined as the temperature at which the pure liquid and solid exist in equilibrium. In practice it is taken as the temperature of the equilibrium mixture at an external pressure of 1 atm; this is sometimes known as the normal freezing or melting point.

The heat absorbed when a gram of a solid melts or the heat liberated when it freezes is known as the latent heat of fusion and for water at 0 °C it is about 80 cal/g (1436 cal/mole). The heat added during the melting process does not bring about a change in temperature until all of the solid has disappeared, since this heat is converted into the potential energy of the molecules that have escaped from the solid into the liquid state.

Changes of the freezing or melting point with pressure may be obtained by using one form of the Clapeyron equation. It is written

$$\frac{\Delta T}{\Delta P} = T\frac{v_l - v_s}{\Delta H_f}$$

where v_l and v_s are the molar volumes of the liquid and solid respectively. Molar volume (vol. in cm^3 per mole) is computed by dividing by gram molecular weight by the density of the compound. ΔH_f is molar heat of fusion, that is the amount of heat absorbed when 1 mole of the solid changes into 1 mole of liquid, and ΔT is the change of melting point brought about by a pressure change of ΔP.

Water is unusual in that it has a lager molar volume in the solid state than in the liquid state ($v_s > v_l$) at the melting point. Therefore, $\Delta T/\Delta P$ is negative, signifying that the melting point is lowered by an increase in pressure. This phenomenon can be rationalised in terms of Lechatelier's principle, which states that a system at equilibrium readjusts so as to reduce the effect of an external stress. Accordingly if a pressure is applied to ice at 0 °C, it will be transformed into liquid water, that is into the state of lower volume, and the freezing point will be lowered.

Hence an increase of pressure of 1 atm lowers the freezing point of water by about 0.0075°, or an increase in pressure of about 133 atm would be required to lower the freezing point of water by1°. Pressure has only a slight effect on the equilibrium temperature of condensed system the large volume or low density of ice accounts for the fact the ice floats on liquid water. The lowering of melting point with increasing pressure is taken advantage of in ice skating. The pressure of the skate lowers the melting point and thus causes the ice to melt below the skate. This thin layer of liquid provides lubricating action allows the skate to state also contributes greatly to the melting and lubricating action.

Melting Point and Intermolecular Forces: The heat of fusion may be considered as the heat required to increase the interatomic or intermolecular distances in crystals, thus allowing melting to occur. A crystal that is bound together by weak forces has a low heat of fusion and a low melting point and crystals which are bound together by strong forces will have a high heat of fusion and high melting points.

Paraffins crystallize as thin leaflets composed of zig-zag chains packed in a parallel arrangement. The melting points of normal saturated hydrocarbons increase with molecular weight because the Vander Waals force between the molecules of the crystal and become greater with an increasing number of carbon atoms. The melting points of the alkanes with an even number of carbon atoms are higher than those of the hydrocarbons with an odd number of carbon atoms. This phenomenon presumably is due to the fact that alkanes with an odd number of carbon atoms are packed in the crystal less efficiently.

The melting points of normal carboxylic acids also show this alteration. This can be explained as follows: fatty acids crystallize in molecular chains. The even carbon acids are arranged in the crystal as seen in the more symmetric structure I, whereas the odd numbered acids are arranged according to structure II. The carboxyl groups are joined together at two points in the even carbon compound; hence the crystal lattice is more stable and the melting point is higher.

The melting points and solubilities of the xanthines of pharmaceutical interest determined by Guttman and Higuchi further exemplify the relationship between melting point and molecular structure. Solubilities like mleting points, are strongly influenced by intermolecular forces. The methylation of theophylline to form caffine and lengthening of the side chain from methyl (caffine) to propyl in the 7th position results in decreases of the melting points and in increase in solubilities. These effects presumably are due to progressive weakening of intermolecular forces.

Polymorphism: Some substances has got the property of existing in different forms. This property is known as polymorphism and the forms are referred to as polymorphs. And if the substance is an element then the property is known as allotropy.

Among the polymorphs some are stable and some are less stable. The less stable forms are known as metastable form. And sometimes the less stable forms are converted in to a stable form and this property is known as monotrophy. Sometimes the polymorphs interchanges between themselves according to the environmental conditions like temperature etc. This property is known as enantiotropy. The temperature at which inter conversion of the poymorphs takes place is known as transition temperature, and the process is known as transition.

Different theories has been proposed to explain the stability of polymorphs. These are based up on different criteria.

1. *Based on Free Energy:* According to this the polymorph with less free energy is referred to as the most stable one.

2. *Heat of Transition Rule:* If the endothermic transition takes place for the given polymorphs then both the polymorphs bear the enantiotrophic relationship at a lower temperature. If these takes place an exothermic transition then the given polymorphs may have a monotrophic relationship or at the temperature higher than the exotherm then they bear an exothermic relationship.

3. Heat of fusion rule.

4. *Density Rule:* The most dense form will be the most stable one at the absolute zero. But this is applied only for the molecular solids where the intra-molecular hydrogen bonding is not significant.

The polymorphs are formed because of the differences in the arrangement of the unit cells. Because of the differences in arrangement, the different properties like heat capacity, conductivity, volume, density, viscosity, surface tension, diffusivity crystal hardness, crystal shape, refractive index, melting or sublimation properties, latent heat of fusion, stability, solubility etc arises in the polymorphs.

As the polymorphs of the same substance has got the different properties it is necessary to study them. The polymorphs have different melting points, x-ray diffraction patterns and solubilities but they are chemically identical.

Generally the property of polymorphism is exhibited by longchain fatty acids because of the attachment difference between the carboxyl groups of adjacent molecules.

Triglyceride tristearin has three forms (three polymorphs)

They are metastable (α) $\rightarrow$ low melting point

Betaprine (β') form

Stable beta (β) form $\rightarrow$ high melting point

The conversion of metastable to stable form takes place but the vice-versa is not possible.

Theobromo oil or cocoabutter is used as a suppositoty base. And it has got four polymorphs. It consists of a single glycerida which has got the narrow temperature range ($34 - 36\,^{\circ}$C). The four polymorphs are:

Unstable gamma $\rightarrow$ m.p. $- 18\,^{\circ}$C

Alpha form $\rightarrow$ m.p. $- 22\,^{\circ}$C $\qquad\Big\}\qquad$ metastable forms

Beta prime form $\rightarrow$ m.p. $- 28\,^{\circ}$C

Stable Beta form $\rightarrow$ m.p $\rightarrow 34.5\,^{\circ}$C $+ \qquad$ stable form

In the preparation of suppository we have to melt the base and it should be poured into the moulds, for that purpose we have to heat it. If we heat the theobromo oil to $35\,^{\circ}$C where it is completely liquefied then the nuclei of the stable form gets destroyed. And it does not crystallize until it is super cooled to $15\,^{\circ}$C. So formed crystals are the metastable forms which melt at 23° to $24\,^{\circ}$C. But such type of bases are not useful for the preparation of suppositories. So we have to heat the theobromo oil to $33\,^{\circ}$C where it will be in a state of liquid which is quite enough to be poured into the moulds. At this state the nuclei of the stable Beta form will also be retained. And after cooling the suppositories are formed which will be having a melting point of $34.5\,^{\circ}$C.

Polymorphs will be having thus different solubilities. If the solubility of drug is less than the rate of dissolution and the bioavailability of drug is also less. For example, chloromphenicol palmiate is very much influenced by this polymorphism.

Sulfameter $\rightarrow$ antibacterial agent $\rightarrow$ form II is more active orally than form III.

Suspension Technology: Cortisone acetate occurs in five different forms. Of these 4 forms are unstable. These will change into a stable polymorph in the presence of water or heating or grinding. Due to this caking of the crystals will be observed due to which the suspension stability will be effected. Because of this reason only before formulating the (emulsion) suspension, cortisone acetate should be in a stable form.

Spiperone (Antipsychotic agent) has got two polymorphs and the arrangement of the crystal or crystal structure of both these polymorphs is different. Polymorph II is made up of dimers. The polymorph I consists of nondimerized molecules.

The difference in the intermolecular Vander Waals forces and hydrogen bonding were found to produce different crystal structures in the antisychotrophic drugs like haloperiodol.

Hydrogen bonding difference led to polymorphism in sulphonamides.

Tamonifen citrate – Antiestrogenic and antineoplastic drug

(used in treatment of breast cancer)

It consists of form A and form B

Form B: it consists of hydrogen bonding which is formed between the carboxyl group of citric acid and the nitrogen of next tamonifen.

Form A: metastable polymorph. But its molecular structure is less organised. Ethanolic suspension of polymorph A rearranges into polymorph B.

Carbamazepines: used in the treatment of epilepsy and trigeminal neuralgia (severe pain in the face, lips and tongue).

β polymorph is crystallised from solvents of high dielectric constant (such as aliphatic alcohols) on the other hand α polymorph is crystallised from solvents of low dielectric constant (e.g., CCl_4 and cyclohexane).

Estrogens are essential hormones for the development of female sex characteristics. When the potent synthetic estrogen, ethyxylestradiol is crystallised from the solvents acetonitrile, methanol, and chloroform saturated with water, four different crystalline solvents formed. Ethxylestradiol has been reported to exist in several polymorphic forms. However, Ishida et. al., have now shown from thermal analysis infrared spectroscopy and x-ray studies that these forms are crystals containing solvent molecules and thus should be classified as solvates rather than as polymorphs. Solvates are sometimes called pseudo polymorphs.

Amorphous Solids: Amorphous solids may be considered as super cooled liquids in which the molecules are arranged in a random manner, somewhat as in the liquid state. Substances such as glass, pitch, and many synthetic plastics are amorphous solids. They differ from crystalline solids in that they tend to flow when subjected to sufficient pressure over a period of time, and they do not have definite melting points.

Amorphous substances as well as cubic crystals, are usually isotropic, that is they exhibit similar properties in all direction. Crystals other than the cubic are anisotrophic, showing different characteristics in various directions along the crystal.

It is not always possible to determine by casual observation whether a substance is crystalline or amorphous. Bees wax and paraffin, although they appear to be amorphous, assume crystalline arrangement when heated and then allowed to cool slowly. Petrolatum as already mentioned, contain both crystalline and amorphous constituents. Some amorphous materials such a glass, may crystallize after long standing.

Whether drug is amorphous or crystalline, it has been shown to affect its therapeutic activity. Thus the crystalline form of the antibiotic novobiocin acid is poorly absorbed and has no activity, whereas the amorphous form is readily absorbed and therapeutically active.

Liquid Crystalline State: The liquid crystal is an apparent contradiction, but it is useful in a descriptive sense since materials in this state are in many ways intermediate between the liquid and solid states.

Structure of Liquid Crystals: Generally molecules in the liquid state are mobile in three directions and can also rotate about three axes perpendicular to one another. On the other hand, in the solid state the molecules are immobile and rotations are not possible.

It is not unreasonable to suppose, therefore that intermediate states of mobility and rotation should exists as in fact they do. It is these intermediate states that constitute the liquid crystalline phase or mesophase as the liquid crystalline phase is called.

The two main types of liquid crystals are termed smectic (soap or grease like) and nematic (thread-like). In the smectic state, molecules are mobile in two direction and can rotate about one axis. In the nematic state, the molecules again rotate only about one axis but mobile in three dimension. A third type (cholesteric crystals) exists but may be considered as a special case of the nematic type.

The smectic mesophase is probably of most pharmaceutical significance since it is this phase that usually forms in ternary (or more complex) mixtures containing a surfactant, water is a weakly amphiphilic or nonpolar-additive.

In general, molecules that form mesophases are organic, are elongated and rectilinear in shape are rigid and posses strong dipoles and easily polarizable groups. The liquid crystalline state any result either from the heating of solids (thermotrophic liquid crystals) or from the action of certain solvents on solids (lyotrophic liquid crystals).

Properties and significance of liquid crystals: Because of their intermediate nature, liquid crystals have some of the properties of liquids and some of solids. For e.g., liquid crystals are mobile and thus can be considered to have the flow properties of liquids. At the same time they possess; the property of being birefringence, the light passing through a material is divided into two components with different velocities and hence different refractive indices.

Some liquid crystals show consistent colour changes with temperature, and this characteristic has resulted in their being used to detect areas of elevated temperature under the skin that may be due to a disease process. Nematic liquid crystals are sensitive to electric fields a property used to advantage in developing display systems. The smectic mesophase has application in the solubilization of water-insoluble materials. It also appears that liquid crystalline phases of this type are frequently present in emulsion and may be responsible for enhanced physical stability owing to their highly viscous nature.

The liquid crystalline state is widespread in nature, with lipoidal form found in nerves, brain tissue, and blood vessels. Atherosclerosis may be related to the laying down of liquid in the liquid crystalline state on the walls of the blood vessels. The three components of bile (cholesterol, a bile acid salt and water) in correct proportions, can form a smectic mesophase, and this may be involved in the formation of gallstones. Bogardus applied the principle of liquid crystal formation to the solubilization and dissolution of cholesterol the major constituent of gallstones. Cholesterol is converted to a liquid crystalline phase in the presence of sodium oleate and water, and the cholesterol, rapidly dissolves from the surface of gallstones.

Non aqueous liquid crystals may be formed from triethanol amine (TEA) and oleic acid with a series of poly ethylene glycols or various organic acids such as isopropyl myristate, squalene, squalene and naphthenic oil as the solvents to replace the water of aqueous mesomorphs. Triangular plots or tetiary phase diagram were used to show that the regions of the liquid crystalline phase when either polar (polyethylene glycols) or nonpolar (squalene) etc compounds were present as a solvent.

Ibrahim studied the release of salicyclic acid as a model drug from hypotrophic liquid crystalline systems a cross lipoidal barriers and into an aqueous buffered solution.

Finally the liquid crystals have structure that are believed to be similar to those in cell membranes. As such liquid crystals may function as useful biophysical models for the structure and functionality of cell membrane.

1.5 Phase Equilibria and the Phase Rule

The condition relating to physical equilibria between various states of matter are conveniently expressed by phase rule. In order to understand this rule, it is first necessary to explain what is meant by the term 'phase', number of components, and 'degrees of freedom'.

Phase (P): A phase is defined as any homogenous and physically distinct part of a system that is separated from other parts of the system by definite boundaries.

e.g., A mixture of gases always constitute one phase because the mixture is homogenous and there are no bounding surfaces between the different gases in the mixture.

No. of Components (C): The no. of components of a system is the smallest no. of independent chemical constituents necessary to express the conc of all phases present in the system.

e.g., In the case of three phase system ice, water and water vapour, the no. of components is one. Since each phase can be expressed in terms of H_2O. A mixture of salt and water is a two component system since both chemical species are independent.

Degrees of Freedom (7): The no. of degrees of freedom is the no. of variable conditions such as temperature, pressure and concentration that it is necessary to state. In order that the condition of the system at equilibrium may be completely define refractive index, density, viscosity etc.

J.Willard tibbs is the person who has formulated the phase rule relating the effect of the least no. of independent variables upon various phases (solid, liquid, gas) that can exist in an equilibrium system containing a given no. of components.

The phase rule is expressed as

$$F = C - P + 2 \quad \text{F-degrees of freedom}$$
$$\text{C-No. of components}$$
$$\text{P-phase}$$

Generally the phase rule is used to define the no. of degrees of freedom that exists for a given system.

E.g., for instance if we consider a gas at a particular temperature then the temperature itself is not sufficient to completely define the system either we must have pressure or other parameters of the system which varies independently with volume regarding to temperature. Then it is clear that this type of system requires two degrees of freedom in order to completely define the system

$$F = 1 - 1 + 2 = 2$$

This is also (proved) confirmed by the phase rule.

Next if we consider a system with water and its vapour then this system can be completely defined by using one variable also became let it be temperature because. The pressure at which the both the phase coexists is also defined

$$F = 1 - 2 + 2 = 1$$

Again this is confirmed by the phase rule.

1.5.1 Systems Containing One Component

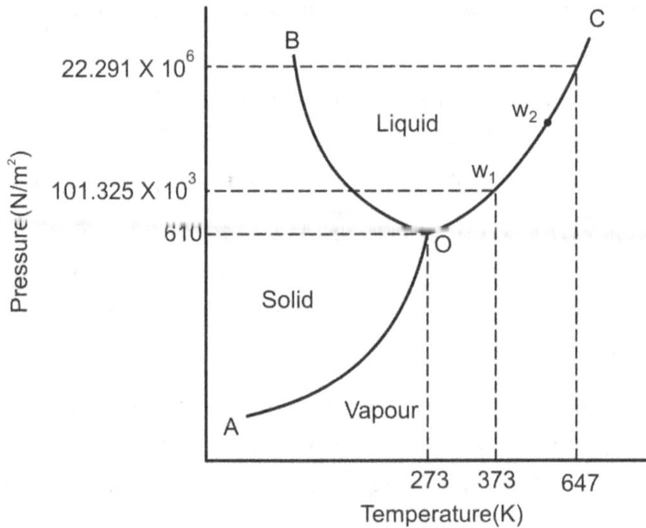

Fig. 1.3 Phase diagram for water at moderate temperature and pressure.

The phase diagram for ice-water-water vapour system may be used to illustrate the interpenetration of these diagrams for one-component system. This particular diagram is also of importance in the understanding the process of freeze drying.

Here in the Fig. 1.3 the areas each correspond to a single phase. The no. of degrees of freedom is given by

$$F = 1 - 1 + 2 = 2$$

This means that temperature and pressure can be varied independently in these areas. For e.g., by varying the temperature and pressure, a mass of water under condition corresponding to point w_1, may be converted to a mass at higher temperature and pressure at point w_2 i.e., this independent variation of temperature and pressure has not altered the no. of phases in the system. However if the conditions are such that the system corresponds to a point that lies on one of the lines AO, BO or CO then two phases now exist in equilibrium with each other, since these lines form the boundaries between different phases. The no. of degrees of freedom is reduced because from eq.

$$F = C - P + 2 \qquad F = 1 - 2 + 2 = 1$$

This means that a single variable exists when equilibrium is established between two phases and if the pressure is altered, the temperature will assume a particular value or conversely if the temperature is altered, the pressure will have a definite value.

Triple Points: The boundary line meet at 'O' which is the only point in the diagram where three phases may coexist in equilibrium and its is therefore termed a triple point. The applications of the phase rule equations to the system at 'O' shows that

$$f = 1 - 3 + 2 = 0$$

The system is therefore invariant, i.e., any change in pressure or temperature will result in an alteration of the no. of phases that are present.

The triple point for water occurs at a temperature of 273.1598 K and a pressure of 610 N/m^2. Thus the triple point temperature is 0.0098 °C above the usual freezing point of water at 1.01325×10^5 N/m^2.

Condensed System: Systems in which the vapour phase is ignored and only solid and/or liquid phases are considered are termed as condensed systems.

Zeotrophic Mixture: Systems where the total vapour pressure is always intermediate between those of the pure components i.e., there is neither as maximum nor minimum in the vapour pressure composition.

e.g., CCl$_4$, Cyclohexane, H$_2$O and Methanol

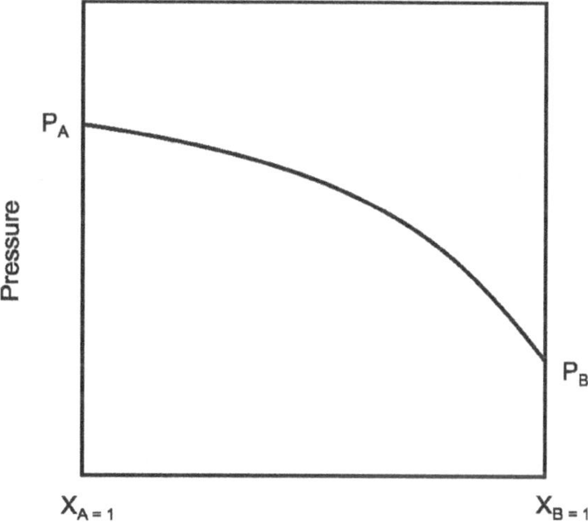

Fig. 1.4

For the purpose of explaining the effects of distillation it is more convenient to use a phase diagram that shows the variation in boiling point with composition of the liquid and vapour phase at constant pressure. It should be observed that the upper and lower curves represent the vapour composition and liquid composition respectively and that the areas corresponding to liquid and vapour phases are transported when compared with the vapour pressure diagrams.

Kon Walff's rule (the vapour pressure in equilibrium with a particular liquid composition is richer in the more volatile component i.e., the component with a higher vapour pressure) can still be seen to apply in the boiling point diagram, since a liquid with a composition corresponding to l_1, will boil at temperature T_1 and be in equilibrium with vapour of composition l_2. This vapour is therefore richer in component A_1 which has the lower boiling point (T_A) and is therefore the more volatile component of the liquid mixture.

If the vapour of composition l_2 is removed and condensed it will give a liquid of composition l_2. If this liquid is subsequently heated it will boil at temperature T_2 to provide a vapour of composition l_3 that is even richer in component A; i.e., the composition of the distillate will approach closer to pure A as more stages of heating and condensation are involved. Conversely as vapour that is richer in A is removed from the distillation flask, the composition of the liquid remaining in the flask gradually approaches pure B. Thus, the components of a zeotrophic mixture may be separated completely by the process of fractional distillation which involves the occurrence of many individual stages of vapourisation and condensation in a distillation column.

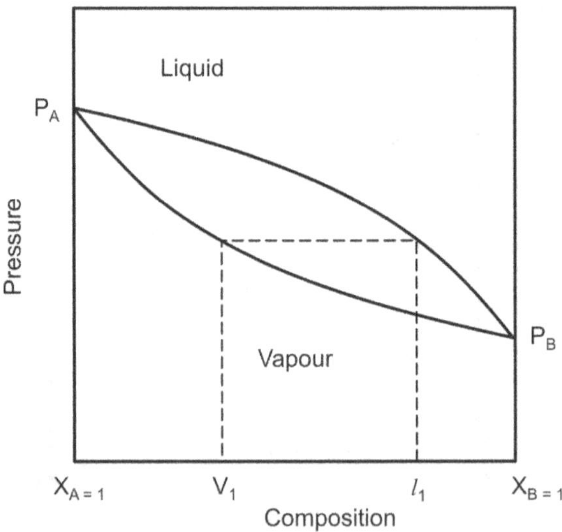

Fig. 1.5 Vapour pressure diagram showing liquid and vapour composition curves (zeotrophic mixture)

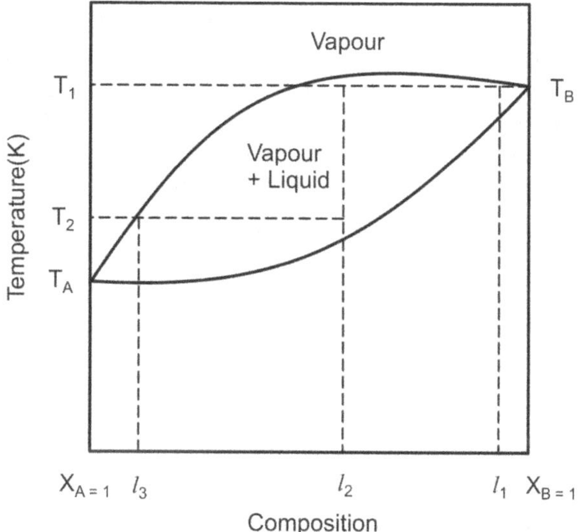

Fig. 1.6 Boiling point composition diagram of a zeotrophic system

If the phase rule is applied to the two component system in the distillation flask where two phase (i.e., liquid and vapour) are present it can be shown that two degrees of freedom exist

$$f = 2 - 2 + 2 = 2$$

Since the pressure is kept constant, the temperature will therefore change as the composition varies in order to maintain the same no. of phase. i.e., the boiling point of the liquid remaining in the flask increases as its composition approaches pure B.

1.5.2 Partially Miscible Liquids

Systems Showing an Increase in Miscibility with Rise in Temperature: A positive deviation from Raoults law arises from a difference in the cohesive forces that exist between the molecules of each component in a liquid mixture. This difference become masked as the temperature decreases, and the positive deviation may then result in a decrease in miscibility sufficient to cause the separation of the mixture into two phases. Each phase consists of a saturated solution of one component in the other liquid. Such mutually saturated solutions are known as conjugated solutions.

The equilibria that occur in mixtures of partially miscible liquid may be followed either by shaking the two liquids together at constant temperature and analysing the samples from each phase after equibrium has been attained, or by observing the temperature at which known proportion of the two liquids contained in the sealed glass ampules become miscible as shown by the disappearance of turbidity.

We know from experience that ethyl alcohol and water are miscible in all proportions, where as water and mercury are for all practical purposes completely immiscible regardless of the relative amounts of each present. Between these two extremes lies a whole range of systems that exhibit partial miscibility (or immiscibility). Such a system is phenol and water and a portion of condensed phase diagram is plotted. The curve gbhci shows the limits of temperature and concentration within which two liquid phases exist in equilibrium. The region outside this curve contains systems having only one liquid phase

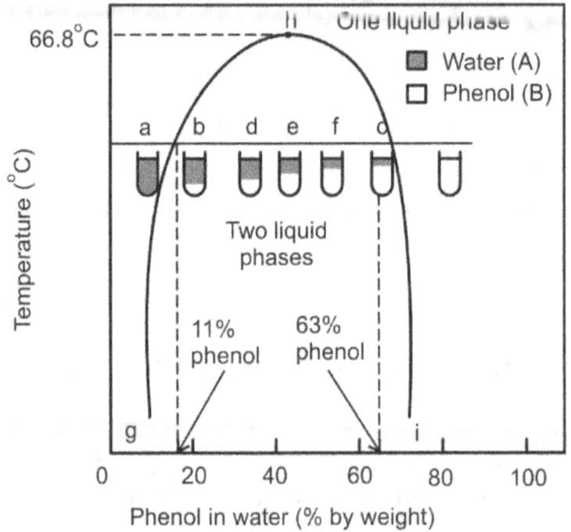

Fig. 1.7 Temperature–composition diagram for the system consisting of water and phenol.

starting at the point a, equivalent to a system containing 100% water (i.e., pure water) at 50 °C, the addition of known increments of phenol to a fixed weight of water, the whole being maintained at 50 °C, will result in the formation of a single liquid phase until the point b is reached at which a minute amount of a second phase appears.

The concentration of phenol and water at which this occurs is 11% by weight of phenol in water. Analysis of the second phase, which separates out on the bottom, show it to contain 63% by weight of phenol in water. This phenol rich phase is denoted by the point C on the phase diagram. As we prepare mixtures containing increasing quantities of phenol, that is as we proceed across the diagram from point b to point c, we form systems in which the amount of the phenol rich phase (B) continually increases as denoted by the test tube. At the same time, the amount of the water rich phase (A) decreases. Once the total concentration of phenol exceeds 63% at 50°, a single phenol-rich liquid phase is formed.

The maximum temperature at which the two phase region exists is termed the critical solution, or upper consolute temperature. In the case of the phenol and water above this temperature are completely miscible and yield one-phase liquid systems.

The line bc drawn across the region containing two phases is termed a tie-line; it is always parallel to the base line in two compound systems. An important feature of phase diagrams is that all systems prepared on a tie line, at equilibrium, will separate into phase of constant composition. These phases are termed conjugate phases. For example, any system represented by a point on the line bc, at 50 °C, seperates to give a pair of conjugate phase whose composition is b and c. The relative amounts of the two layers or phases vary. Thus if we prepare a system containing 24% by weight of phenol and 76% by weight of water (point d) at equilibrium we have two liquid phases present in the tube. The upper one A, has a composition of 11% phenol in water (point b or the diagram) while the lower layer, B, contains 63% phenols (point C on the diagram). Phase B will lie below phase A since it is rich in phenol and phenol has a higher density than water. In term of the relative weights of the two phases, there will be more of the water-rich phase A then the phenol-rich phase B at point f.

Thus,

$$\frac{\text{Weight of phase A}}{\text{Weight of phase B}} = \frac{\text{Length dc}}{\text{Length bd}}$$

The right hand term might appear at first glance to be the reciprocal of the proportion one should write. The weight of phase A is greater than phase B, however became point d is closer to point b than it is to point c. The lengths dc and bd can be measured with a rules in centimetres or inches from the phase diagram, but it is frequently more convenient to use the units of percent weight of phenol on the abscissa. For e.g., since point b = 11%, point c = 63% and point d = 24%, the ratio dc/bd = (63 – 24)/ (24 – 11) = 39/13 = 3/1. In other words, for every 10 gm of a liquid system in equilibrium represented by point d, one finds 7.5 gm of phase A and 2.5 gm of phase B. If, on the other hand, we prepare a system containing 50% by weight of phenol (point f), the ratio phase A to phase B = fc/bf = (63 – 50)/(50 – 11) = 13/39 = 1/3. Accordingly for every 10 gm of system f prepared, we obtain an equilibrium mixture of 2.5 gm of phase A and 7.5 gm of phase B. It should be apparent that a system containing 37% by weight of phenol will under equilibrium conditions at 50 °C, give equal weights of phase A and phase B.

Working on a tie line in a phase diagram enables us to calculate the composition of each phase in addition to the weight of the phases. Thus, it becomes a simple matter to calculate the distribution of phenol (or water) through out the system as a whole. As an example let us suppose that we mixed 24 gm of phenol with 76 gm of water, warmed the mixture to 50 °C, and allowed it to reach equilibrium at this temperature. On separation of the two phases, we would find 75 gm of phase A (containing 11% by weight of phenol) And 25gm of phase B (containing 63% by weight if phenol). Phase A therefore contains a total of (11 × 75)/100 = 8.25 gm of phenol, while phase B contains a total of (63 × 25)/100 = 15.75 gm of phenol. This gives a sum total of 24 gm of phenol in the whole system. This equals the amount of phenol originally added and therefore confirm our assumptions and calculations. It is left to the reader to confirm that phase A contains 66.75 gm of water and phase B 9.25 gm of water.

Phenol and water system has got many pharmaceopeal applications. Some of the other combinations are water-aniline, carbon-disulphide-methyl alcohol, isopentane-phenol methyl alcohol-cyclohexane and isobutyl alcohol-water.

Some of the mixtures consists of lower consolute temperatures below which both the liquids are miscible in all proportion e.g., for that type of system is triethylamine-water system.

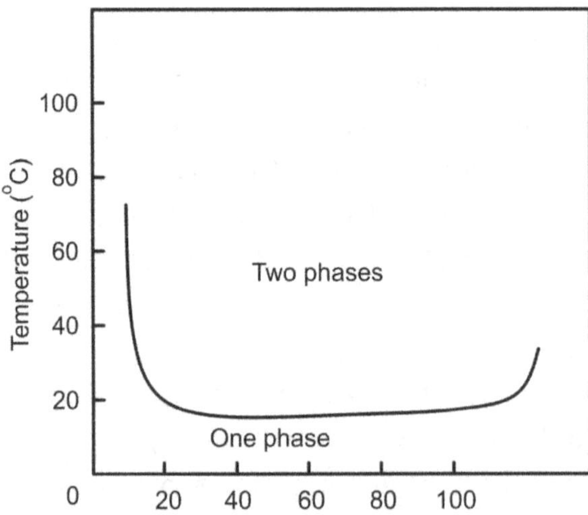

Fig. 1.8 Phase diagram for the system triethylamine – water showing lower consolute temperature.

Some of the mixtures shows both lowers and upper consolute temperature.

e.g., nicotine-water system

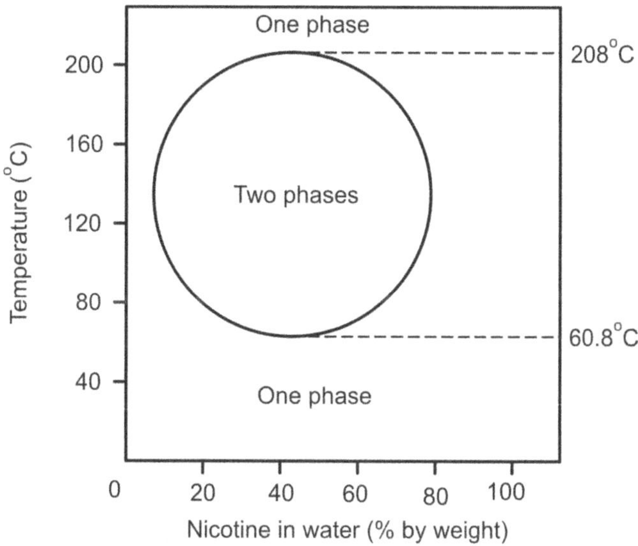

Fig. 1.9 Nicotine-water system showing upper and lower consolute temperature.

Two component systems containing solids and liquids phases. The behaviours of two component solid-liquid systems can e classified into three types.

1. Systems that show the formation of a Eutectic mixture.
2. Systems that show the formation of a compound with a congruent melting point (i.e., the compound which consists of one component solvated by the other, yields a liquid with the same composition as the compound on mleting).
3. Systems that show the formation of a compound with an incongruent melting point i.e., the compound undergoes fusion on heating to a certain temperature and produces a liquid and a new solid phase, the composition of which is different from that of the original compound.

System of the first type, which involve the formation of a eutectic mixture, have found certain applications of pharmaceutical interest. The other types are of less importance.

1.5.3 Formation of Eutectic Mixtures

The ice-kcl system shows the behaviour of a entectic mixture.

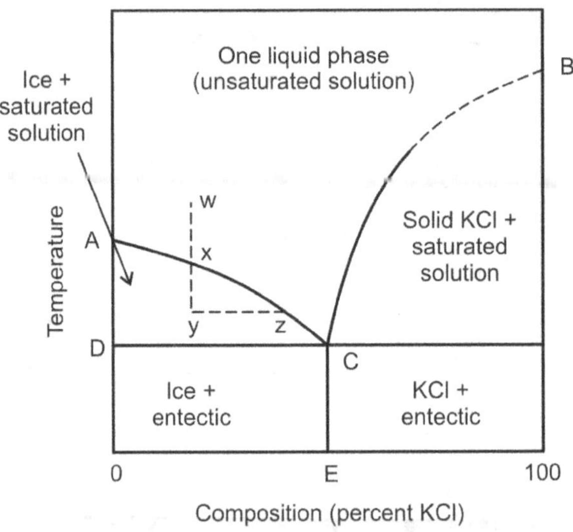

Fig. 1.10 Temperature composition diagram for the KCl-water system.

Here A and B represent the meting points of ice and kcl respectively. If KCl is added to water, the freezing point of the latter is reduced as indicated by AC, which therefore represents the effect of composition on the temperature at which ice separates from the system. Similarly if water is added to KCl the melting point of the latter is lowered, BC therefore represents the effect of composition on the temperature at which solid KCl separates from the system.

At C, both solid components can exist in equilibrium, with a liquid of definite composition. Application of the 'reduced phase rule' shows that the system is invariant at this point since there are no degrees of freedom

$$f' = 2 + 1 - 3 = 0$$

This means that the mixture will freeze completely at a constant temperature D, which is lower than the freezing points of either pure component.

Further understanding of the phase diagram may be obtained by considering the effect of cooling a solution of KCl in water represented by point w in the diagram. If the solution is cooled to point x on the freezing curve AC, then some ice will separate out. Further cooling to y will produce more ice and the remaining solution will become more concentrated since it will contain all the original KCl. The composition of the remaining solution will correspond to point z. As the temperature falls, the composition of the remaining liquid moves along AC. A limit is reached when the remaining solution is saturated with kcl and on cooling this solution ice and KCl will seperate out in the same ratio in which they exist in the saturated solution has solidified. The mixture, which separates at this temperature termed as eutectic (or a cryohydrate, if one of the components is water) and its composition is given by E. Although the eutectic has a definite melting point, the following evidence suggests that it is an intimate mechanical mixture and not a compound.

(a) The components can be separated mechanically

(b) The addition of each component raises the melting point of the eutectic. The melting point of a compound would be lowered on admixture with another substance.

(c) A heterogeneous structure can be seen under a microscope

(d) X-ray analysis reveals the existence of two phases.

The areas in the phase diagram each correspond to the existence of various phases or mixtures of phases.

The phase-diagram for the water-KCl system may be used to explain the principle of freezing mixture prepared from ice and salt. If salt is added to ice and a little water, some of the salt will dissolve in the water to produce a system composed of ice, salt and solution. Such a system II in stable equilibrium at the eutectic point only. The system will therefore tend to move towards this point and ice will melt and salt will continue to dissolve in the resultant water. Both of these processes are accompanied by absorption of heat and the temperature therefore falls until one of the solid components has been used up completely. If the initial proportion of ice and salt are chosen satisfactory the eutectic temperature will be reached.

It has been suggested that eutectic mixtures may be useful as a means of increasing the rates of solution of slowly soluble drugs in a aqueous body fluids. It was thought that the rapid solution of the second component (e.g., urea in eutectic fine crystalline form that would be more rapidly in a very fine crystalline form that would be more rapidly soluble than the usual forms of the drug. However subsequent studies have suggested that this increased dissolution rates of the drugs in the presence of urea is likely to be caused by the formation of solid solutions of these drugs with urea and not by eutectic formation.

1.5.4 Phase Equilibria in Three Component Systems

In systems containing three components but only one phase $f = 3 - 1 + 2 = 4$ for a noncondensed system. The four degrees of freedom are temperature, pressure and the concentration of two of the three components. Only two concentration terms are required became the sum of these substracted from the total will give the concentration of the third component. If we regard the system as condensed and hold the temperature constant then

F = 2 and we can again use a plane diagram to illustrate the phase equilibria, because we are dealing with a three component system. It is more convenient to use triangular coordinate graphs, although it is possible to use rectangular co-ordinates.

The various phase equilibria that exist in three-component systems containing liquid and/or solid phases are frequently complex. Certain typical three-component systems are discussed here, however, because they are of pharmaceutical interest, for example, several areas of pharmaceutical processing such as crystallization, salt form selection, and chromatographic analyses rely on the use of terenary systems for optimization.

Rules Relating to Triangular Diagrams

Before discussing phase equilibria interenary systems, it is essential that the reader become familiar with certain rules that relate to the use of triangular co-ordinates. It should have been apparent in discussing two component systems that all concentrations were expressed on a weight-weight basis this is because, although it is an easy and direct method of preparing dispersion, such an approach also follows the concentration to be expressed in terms of the mole fraction or the molality. The concentration in ternary systems are accordingly expressed on a weight basis.

1. Each of the three corners of apexes of the triangle represent 100% by weight of one component (A, B or C). As a result that same apex will represent 0% of the other two components.

2. The three lines joining the corner points represent two component mixtures of the three possible combinations of A, B, and C. Thus the lines AB, BC and CA are used for two component mixtures of A and B, B and C, and C and A respectively. By dividing each line into 100 equals units, we can directly relate the location of a point along the line to the percent concentration of one component in a two component system. For e.g., point y midway between A and B on the line AB, represents a system containing 50% of B (and hence 50% of A also) point z, three fourths of the way along BC, signifies a system containing 75% of c in B.

   In goining along a line bounding the triangle so as to represent the concentration in a two components system, it does not maters whether we proceed in a clockwise or a counter clock rise direction around the triangle provided we are consistent. The move usual convention is clockwise and have been adopted here. Hence as we move along AB in the direction of B, we are signifying systems of A and B containing increasing concentrations of B and correspondingly smaller amounts of A. moving along BC toward C will represent systems of B and C containing more and more of C; the closer we approache A on the line CA the greater will be the concentration of A in systems of A and C.

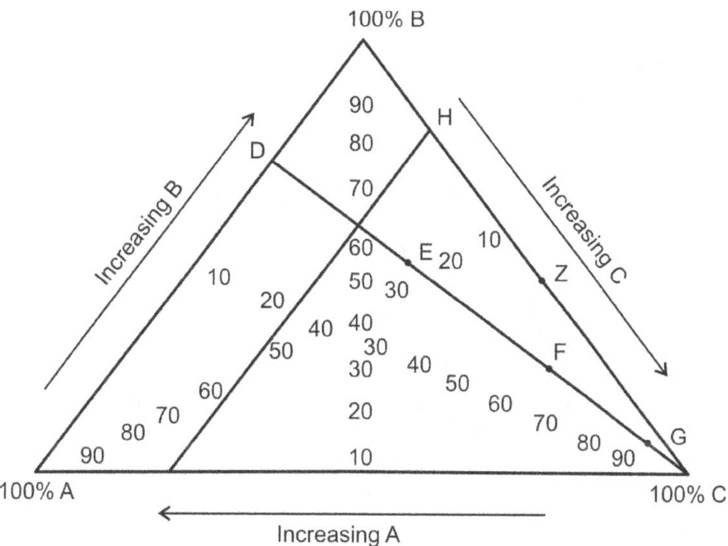

Fig. 1.11 Triangular diagram for three component system.

3. The area within the triangle represents all the possible combinations of A, B, and C to give three component systems. The location of x particular three component system within the triangle for e.g., point can be undertaken as follows:

The line AC opposite apex B represents systems containing A and C component B is absent that is B = 0. The horizontal lines running across the triangle parallel to AC denote increasing percentages of B from B = 0 (on line AC) to B = 100 (at point B), the line parallel to AC that cuts point x is equivalent to 15% B, consequently the systems contains 15% of B and 85% of A and C together. Applying similar arguments to the other two components in the system, we can say that along the line AB, C = 0. As we proceed from the line AB towards across the diagrams C the concentration of C increase until at the apex C = 100%. The point x lies on the line parallel to AB that is equivalent to 30% of C. It follows therefore that the concentration of A is 100 − (B + C) = 100 − (15 + 30) = 55%. This is readily confirmed by proceeding across the diagram from the line BC towards apex A; point x lies on the line equivalent to 55% of A.

4. If a line is drawn through any apex to a point on the opposite side, then all the systems represented by points on. Such a line have a constant ratio of two components in this case A and B. Further more, the continual addition of C to a mixture of A and B will produce systems that lie progressively closer to apex C (100% of component C).

5. Any line drawn parallel to one side of the triangle for example line HI represents ternary system in which the proportion (or percent by weight) of one component is constant. In this instance all systems prepared along HI will contain 20% of C and varying concentration of A and B.

1.5.5 Terenary System with One Pair of Partially Miscible Liquids

Water and benzene are miscible only to a slight extent and so a mixture of the two usually produces a two phase system. The heavier of the two phases consists of water saturated with benzene while the lighter phase is benzene saturated with H_2O. On the other hand, alcohol is completely miscible with both benzene and water. It is to be expected therefore that the addition of sufficient alcohol to a two phase system of C_4H_6 and H_2O would produce a single liquid phase in which all three components are miscible. It might be helpful to consider the alcohol as acting in a manner comparable to that of temperature in the binary phenol-water system considered earlier. Raising the temperature of the phenol-water system led to complete miscibiling of the two conjugate phases and the formation of one liquid phase. The addition of alcohol to the benzene-water system achieves the same end but by different means, namely a solvent effect in place of a temperature effect. There is a strong similarity between the use of heat to break cohesive forces between molecules and the use of solvent to achieve the same result. The effect of alcohol will better understood when we introduce dielectric constant of solutions and solvent in later chapters. In this case alcohol serves as an intermediate polar solvent that shifts the electronic equilibrium of a diametrically opposed highly polar water and nonpolar benzene solutions to provide salvation.

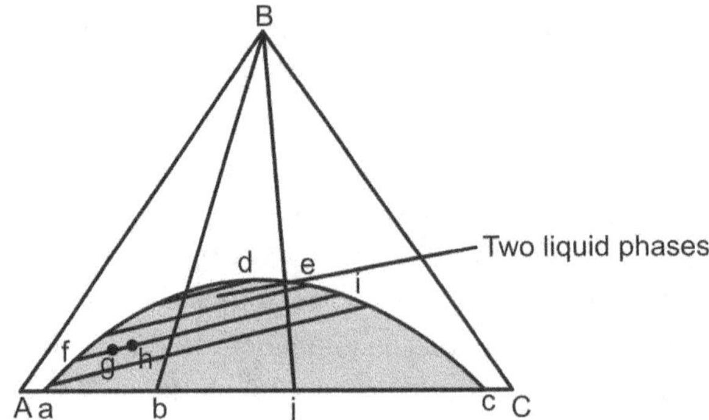

Fig. 1.12 System of three liquids, one pair of which is partially miscible.

Let us suppose that A, and B and C represent water, alcohol and benzene respectively. The line AC therefore depicts bindary mixtures of A and C and the points a and c are the limits of solubility of C in A and of A in C respectively at the particular temperature being used. The curve afdeic frequency termed a binodal or binodal, marks curve or binodal, marks the extent of the phase region. The remainder of the triangle contains one liquid phase. The tie lines within the binodal are not necessarily parallel to one another or to the base line, AC as was the case in the two phase region of binary system. In fact the directions of the tie lines are related to the shape of the binodal which in turn depends on the relative solubility of the third component (in this case, alcohol) in the other two components. Only when the added component acts equally on the other two components to bring them into solution will the bionodal be perfectly symmetric and the tie line run parallel to the base line.

The properties of tie lines discussed earlier still apply and system g and h prepared along the tie line fi both give rise to two phases having the composition denoted by the points f and i. The relative amounts by weight of the two conjugate phase will depend on the position of the original system along the tie line. For e.g., system g after reaching equilibrium will separate into two phases f and i; the ratio of phase f to phases on a weight basis is given by the ratio gi is fg. Mixture h, halfway along the tie line, will contain equal weights of the two phases at equilibrium.

The phase equilibria depicted here show that the addition of component B to a 50:50 mixture of components A and C will produce a phase change from a two liquid system to a one-liquid system at point d, with a 25:75 mixture of A and C shown as point j; the addition of B leads to a phase change at point e. Naturally all mixtures lying along dB and eB will be one phase systems.

As we saw earlier f = 2 in a single-phase region and so we must defined two concentration to fix the particular system. Along the binodal curve afdeic F = 1 and we need to know only one concentration term because this will allows the composition of one phase to be fixed on the binodal curve from the tie line, we can obtain the composition of the conjugate phase.

1.6 Questions

1. Write a short notes on Hydrogen Bonding.

2. What is polymorphism. Give its application in Pharmacy.

3. With the help of a neat labelled diagram explain the phase diagram of phenol water system. How is the tie line useful in calculating the composition of the conjugate layers.

4. Describe the principle involved in aerosols as gaseous dosage forms.

5. List out the different binding forces between the molecules.

6. Write about heat of vaporisation and Heat of a reaction.

7. Mention and explain the important postulates of kinetic molecular theory.

CHAPTER 2

THERMODYNAMICS

2.1 Introduction

The word "Thermodynamics" literally means flow of heat. The term thermodynamics is made up of two words – 'thermo' means heat – 'dynamics' means 'motion' leading to mechanical work. It deals with the energy changes accompanying all types of physical and chemical processes.

The study of thermodynamics is based on three generalisation called First, Second and Third law of thermodynamics. All these laws are based on human experience and there is no formal proof for these laws, but nothing contrary is found against to these laws.

These laws of thermodynamics can be applied only to the "macroscopic" observable properties of matter such as pressure, temperature, volume etc; not to individual atoms (or) molecules and it took about 500 years to establish these laws.

It mainly deals with the transformation of heat into other forms of energy such as mechanical, chemical, electrical and variant energy and vice verse. Thus thermodynamics may now be defined as "branch of science that deals with the quantitative relationships between heat and other forms of energy".

Note: It deals only with the energy changes accompanying a given process (physical (or) chemical) but not the total energy of the body.

34

2.2 Importance of Thermodynamics

- In physics phenomena such as diffusion, complexation, interfacial phenomenon etc. solution, kinetics etc. proceeds with the change in the energy and hence these thermodynamics laws can be used to understand those processes and also to derive various equations relating temperature, vapour pressure, heat of vapourisation and solution processes.

- Regarding chemistry it helps in predicting the feasibility of a particular process (physical or chemical) i.e. whether the process can occur or not under a given set of conditions like temperature, pressure, concentration etc.

- Regarding engineering it helps to know the efficiency of various types of heat engines.

Thus, 'thermodynamics' have many wide spread applications in our day-to-day life hence it is important to have a well knowledge about it.

Limitations of Themodynamics

(i) The laws of the thermodynamics can be applied only to the "macroscopic system" i.e. mater in bulk but not to individual molecules or atoms

(ii) It give no information about the rate at which a given a process may proceed. i.e. it can provide no information about the time taken to reach equilibrium but can tell only about feasibility, direction and extent of a given process.

(iii) It deals only with initial and final state of a system ignoring the path or mechanism of a process.

Definitions of Terms used in Thermodynamics

System and Surroundings:

System may be defined as that part of the universe (i.e. part of matter) under consideration. The remaining part of the universe excluding the system is known as surroundings:

For example, if you are studying about a chemical reaction in a beaker then that beaker and its constituents makes the system and all other objects and portion around that are surroundings of the system.

Note: The walls of the beaker constitute the boundary between the system and surroundings.

Types of Systems:

(i) *Isolated system:* A system in which neither matter nor energy can be exchanged with the surroundings is called isolated system (Fig. 2.1).

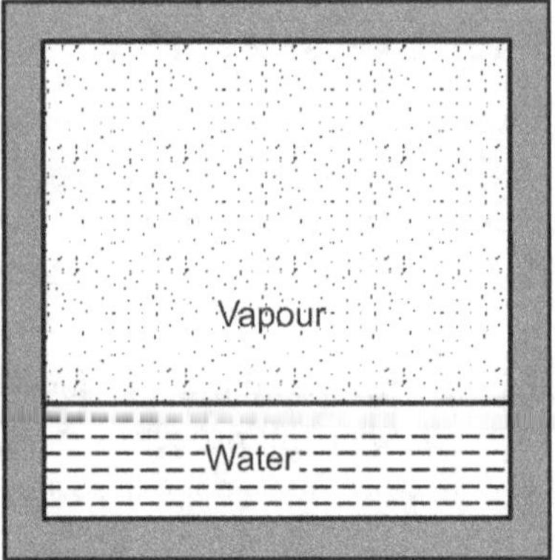

Fig. 2.1 An isolated system.

Consider a beaker with water and its vapour whose walls are insulated. In this the vapour (i.e. matter) can not leave the beaker since it is a closed one and heat too cannot escape due to insulation, hence it can be taken as isolated system.

(ii) *Open system:* A system which can exchange both matter as well as energy with its surroundings is called an open system (Fig. 2.3).

A beaker of water kept in open sun where water vapour (matter) escapes with the absorption of heat energy form surrounds.

(iii) *Closed system:* A system which can exchange energy but not matter with its surroundings is called a closed system (Fig. 2.2).

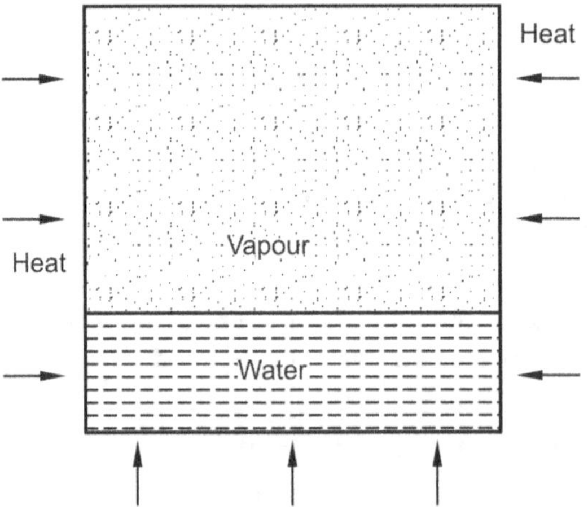

Fig. 2.2 closed system.

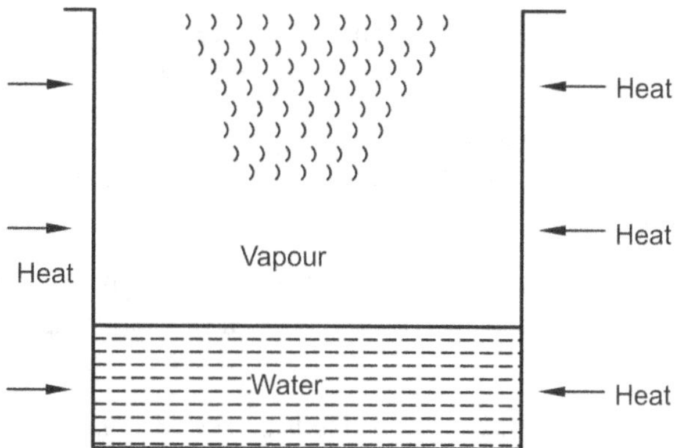

Fig. 2.3 An open system.

Water and its vapour present in an uninsulated beaker where only exchange of heat takes place but not matter due to closed vessel.

Reversible and Irreversible Processes

A reversible process is that which is infinitesimally slowly to that all changes occurring in the direct process can be exactly reversed and the system remains almost in a state of equilibrium at all times.

In another way

It may be defined as that which is carried out in stages and the driving force at every stage is only infinitesimally greater than the opposing force and which can be reversed by increasing the opposing force by an infinitesimal amount.

In order to understand this let us see an experiment.

Consider a cylinder provided with a frictionless piston enclosing a gas, up on which a pile of sand is kept.

The pressure 'p' exerted by the gas on the piston is equal to combined pressure exerted by the weight of the piston, the pile of sand and the atmospheric pressure. Under these conditions since equal pressure is exerted on both sides the piston neither move upwards nor downwards, and there will be no change in the volume.

Suppose a grain of sand is removed, then the pressure on the piston is lowered by infinitesimally small amount (dp) then the pressure on the piston becomes, $\rho - dp$ which is infinitesimally smaller than pressure of the gas 'p' hence the piston moves upwards and the gas expands but in a very small amount. But if suppose a grain of sand is replaced then the gas will return to its original volume.

If suppose the sand particles are continually removed one by one, the gas will expand bit by bit in a very small amount and attains equilibrium in each step.

But if the pressure on the piston is decreased all of a sudden in a single step, the gas will expand suddenly, the volume of the gas increase all of a sudden and it is said to be irreversible expansion.

Therefore now we can define irreversible process as the process which is not carried out in infinitesimally slow steps (instead it is carried out in a single step) and cannot be carried in a reverse order.

All spontaneous processes occurring around us like expansion of gases, flow of heat from hot bodies to cold bodies are irreversible.

Difference between Reversible and Irreversible Process.

(i)	A reversible process takes place slowly in infinite number of infinitesimal in a small steps	(i)	An irreversible process takes place in one rapid measurable step
(ii)	A reversible process is unreal since frictionless and weightless pistons are involved	(ii)	It is a real process and can be performed actually
(iii)	A reversible process is in equilibrium at all stages of the operation	(iii)	It is in equilibrium only at the initial and final stages of the operation
(iv)	It is bi-directional in nature	(iv)	It proceeds only in one direction
(v)	Work done in a reversible process in greater than irreversible	(v)	Work done in this process is less than that of reversible process.

Macroscopic System and Macroscopic Properties:

A system with a large number of particles (molecules, atoms, ions etc.) is known as macroscopic system:

The properties that are concerned with such system are called macroscopic properties.

Ex: Volume, temperature, viscosity, density etc.

Extensive Properties

A property that depends up on the quantity of the substance or substance present in the system is called extensive property.

Ex: Mass, volume

Note: The extensive properties are 'additive' i.e. the total value of extensive property is equal to the sum of the values for the separate parts into which the system is divided.

Intensive Property: A property which depends only up on the nature of the substance and not on the amount of the substance present in the system.

Ex: Temperature, refractive index, specific heat, pressure etc.

Thermodynamic Process

The process by which a thermodynamic system changes from one state to another is called thermodynamic process. Depending up on condition of change, five different types of thermodynamic systems are recognized.

Isothermal Process: A process in which the heat enters or leaves the system but the temperature of the system remains constant throughout the process.

An isothermal reaction may be carried out by placing the system in a large constant – temperature bath so; the heat is drawn or returned to it without affecting the temperature of the system.

$\therefore$ for an isothermal process change in temperature

$$dT = 0$$

Adiabatic Process: A process during which no heat enters or leaves the system during any step of the process is known as adiabatic process.

A reaction carried out in thermally insulated Dewar flask or vacuum bottle is adiabatic.

In this process since no heat enters or leaves the system, the temperature will decrease or increase.

$\therefore$ For adiabatic process change in heat (dq) = 0

$$dq = 0$$

Isobaric Process: A process during which pressure of the system remains constant throughout the reaction is known as isobaric process.

Ex: At boiling point of water its vapourisation takes place at same atmospheric pressure

$\therefore$ For isobaric process

$$dp = 0$$

Isochoric Process: A process during which volume of the system remains constant throughout the reaction is known as isochoric process.

$\therefore$ For isochoric process

$$dv = 0$$

Cyclic Process: A process during which the system comes to its initial state through a number of different processes is called a cycle or cyclic process.

$\therefore$ For cyclic process $dE = 0$

$$dH = 0$$

2.3 First Law of Thermodynamics

- The first law of thermodynamics is simply the law of conservation of energy which states that:

"Energy can neither be created nor destroyed but it can be converted from one form to another".

i.e. the total energy of a system and its immediate surrounding remains constant during any operation. From this we can say that when one kind of energy is formed, an equal amount of another kind will disappear.

According to first law the effect of 'Q' and 'W' in a given system during change of state from initial to final are related to an intrinsic property of the system called Internal energy.

Suppose the system while undergoing change form initial state A [with internal energy E_A] to final state B (with internal energy E_B) absorbs heat Q from the surroundings and performs some work 'W'.

The heat absorbed increase the energy of system and the work done tends to lower the energy of system

$\therefore$ Change in internal energy ΔE can be written as

$$\Delta E = E_2 - E_1 = Q + W \qquad \qquad .....(2.1)$$

- This equation tells us that the work and heat are the equivalent ways of changing the internal energy of the system. By using the eq. (2.1) one can calculate the change in the internal energy by measuring 'Q' and 'W' during change of state.

For an infinitesimal change (small change) in the energy the eq. (2.1) can be written as

$$dE = dq + dw \qquad \qquad .....(2.2)$$

where

dq = heat absorbed, dw = work done during the small change of system

but capital letters Q and W are used for heat and work in eq (2.1) to signify, finite changes in these quantities.

- It is useful to express the change in internal energy in terms of measurable properties of the system P, V and T. By knowing any two of these variable, we can know the internal energy of the system.

- The small change of any state property like dE can also be written as a function of T and V as in the following equation for a closed system [i.e. constant mass]

$$dE = \left(\frac{\partial E}{\partial T}\right)_v dT + \left(\frac{\partial E}{\partial v}\right)_T dv \qquad \ldots\ldots(2.3)$$

This eq. (2.3) tells us about the rate of change in energy with the change in T at constant volume $\left[\left(\frac{\partial E}{\partial T}\right)_v dT\right]$ or with the change of V at constant temperature $\left[\left(\frac{\partial E}{\partial v}\right)_T dv\right]$.

$\therefore$ We can express this eq. in terms of measurable properties by combining eqs. (2.2) and (2.3) into

$$dq + dw = dE = \left(\frac{\partial E}{\partial T}\right)_v dT + \left(\frac{\partial E}{\partial v}\right)_T dv \qquad \ldots\ldots(2.4)$$

2.3.1 Changes of State at Constant Volume

In a process if the volume is kept constant i.e. $dv = 0$, first law can be expressed as

$$dE = dQ_v \qquad \ldots\ldots(2.5)$$

[dE = dQ + dw (eq. 2.2) but we know dw = p.dv

$\therefore \qquad$ dE = dQ + p.dv

But $\qquad$ dv = 0

$\therefore \qquad$ dE = dQ + 0 $\Rightarrow$ dE = dQ$_v$]

where subscript 'v' denotes constant volume.

$\therefore$ At constant volume increase in internal energy of an ideal gas

$$= \text{heat absorbed at constant volume}$$

Heat evolved at constant volume (Q_v) = decrease in internal energy

In short $\qquad \Delta E = Q_v$

- Under these conditions the combined eq. (2.4) is reduced to

$$dq_v = \left(\frac{\partial E}{\partial T}\right)_v dT \qquad \qquad .....(2.6)$$

It tells us about the heat transferred during the process at constant volume (dQ_v) with the change in temperature (dT) and the ratio between these two quantities gives the molar heat capacity at constant volume

$$\overline{C}_v = \frac{dq_v}{dT} = \left(\frac{\partial E}{\partial T}\right)_v \qquad \qquad .....(2.7)$$

where $\overline{C}_v$ = molar heat capacity

Note: "Heat capacity" may be defined as the ratio of the amount of heat absorbed to rise in temp.

2.3.2 Change of State at Constant Pressure

Concept of Enthalpy or Heat Content

- When the work of expansion is done at constant pressure

work done, $\qquad \qquad W = -P\Delta V \qquad \qquad .....(2.8)$

$$= -P(V_2 - V_1)$$

Under these conditions first law becomes

$$\Delta E = Q_p - P\,(V_2 - V_1) \qquad \qquad .....(2.9)$$

where Q_p is the heat absorbed at constant pressure

Now, rearranging the eqn. 2.9

$$Q_p = E_2 - E_1 + P(V_2 - V_1)$$

$$= (E_2 + PV_2) - (E_1 + PV_1) \qquad \qquad .....(2.10)$$

Then the term $E + PV$ gives the "ENTHALPY" (H).

These two factors (internal energy and work function) when combined together gives rise to enthalpy (or) heat content.

Mathematically it is defined by eqn.

$$H = E + PV \qquad \qquad .....(2.11)$$

Thus the eq. (2.10) can be written as follows

$$Q_p = H_2 - H_1 = \Delta H \qquad \qquad .....(2.12)$$

The increase in enthalpy (ΔH) is equal to the heat absorbed at constant pressure by the system and writing eq. (2.11) as

$$\Delta H = \Delta E + P\,\Delta V \qquad\qquad .....(2.13)$$

For an infinitesimal change,

$$dq_p = dH \qquad\qquad .....(2.14)$$

Now Function 'H' can be expressed in the form of variables

$$dH = \left(\frac{\partial E}{\partial T}\right)_p dT + \left(\frac{\partial E}{\partial P}\right)_T dp \qquad\qquad .....(2.15)$$

When the pressure is held constant

$$dH = \left(\frac{\partial H}{\partial T}\right)_p dT \qquad\qquad .....(2.16)$$

Since $dq_p = dH$ at constant pressure according to eq. (2.14) the molar heat capacity C_p at constant pressure

$$\overline{C}_p = \frac{d_{qp}}{dT} = \left(\frac{\partial H}{\partial T}\right)_p \qquad\qquad .....(2.17)$$

For change in Enthalpy between products and reactants

$$\Delta H = H_{products} - H_{reactor}$$

Eq. (2.17) may be written

$$\left[\frac{\partial(\Delta H)}{\partial T}\right]_p = \Delta C_p \qquad\qquad .....(2.18)$$

where $DC_p = (C_p)_{products} - (C_p)_{reactants}$ and the eq. is known as Kirchoff equation.

Work of Exapnsion Against a Constant Pressure

In this case, let us see about the work done against a constant opposing external pressure P_{ext}.

For this imagine a hypothetical cylinder with a Weightless, frictionless Piston of Area 'A' as shown in Fig. 2.4.

If a constant external pressure P_{ext} is exerts on the piston the total force exerted on the piston is given by:

$$\text{Pressure} = \frac{\text{Force}}{\text{Area}}$$

$$\therefore \qquad \text{Force} = P_{ext} \times \text{Area}$$

Now, the vapour in the cylinder is made to expand by increasing the temperature and the piston moves a distance 'h'. Then the work done against the opposing pressure in one single stage is

$$W = -P_{ext} \times A \times h \ [\text{Work} = \text{Force} \times \text{displacement}] \quad \ldots\ldots(2.19)$$

Then $A \times h$ is the increase in volume

$$\Delta V = V_2 - V_1$$

So, that at constant pressure

$$W = -P_{ext} \Delta V = -P_{ext} (V_2 - V_1)$$

$$= -PdV \quad (\text{eq. 2.8})$$

Maximum Work

The work done by a system in an isothermal expansion process is maximum when it is done reversibly. It can be proved by following discussion (Fig. 2.5).

If an ideal gas expands freely into a vacuum, then since no external pressure $(P = 0)$ is present work done is zero

$$W = 0 \times dV$$

$$W = 0$$

If the external pressure is slowly increased, the amount of work done is also increased and it reaches to maximum when the external pressure is infinitesimally less than the pressure of the gas.

If the external pressure is continually increased, the gas is compressed then work is done on the system rather than by the system in an isothermal reversible process.

Then the maximum work done for a system that is expanding in reversible fashion is

$$W = \int_1^2 dw = \int_{V_1}^{V_2} Pdv \ \{P_{ext} \text{ replaced by P}\} \quad \ldots\ldots(2.20)$$

According to ideal gas

$$P = \frac{nRT}{V}$$

Since it is an isothermal process 'T' is constant then 'nRT' becomes constant

$$\therefore \quad W_{max} = \int_{1}^{2} dw_{max} = -nRT \int_{V_1}^{V_2} \frac{dV}{V} \qquad \qquad .....(2.21)$$

Applying log we get

$$W_{max} = -nRT\, ln\, \frac{V_2}{V_1} \qquad \qquad .....(2.22)$$

Applying boyle's law $\dfrac{V_2}{V_1} = \dfrac{P_1}{P_2}$

$$W_{max} = -nRT\, ln\, \frac{P_1}{P_2} \qquad \qquad .....(2.23)$$

The eq. (2.20) not only gives the maximum work done but it also tells the minimum work done, when the gas is reversibly compressed and when the P_{ext} is only infinitesimally larger than P.

The Fig. 2.5 shows the area representing the "maximum expansion work" or the "minimum compression work" in a reversible process.

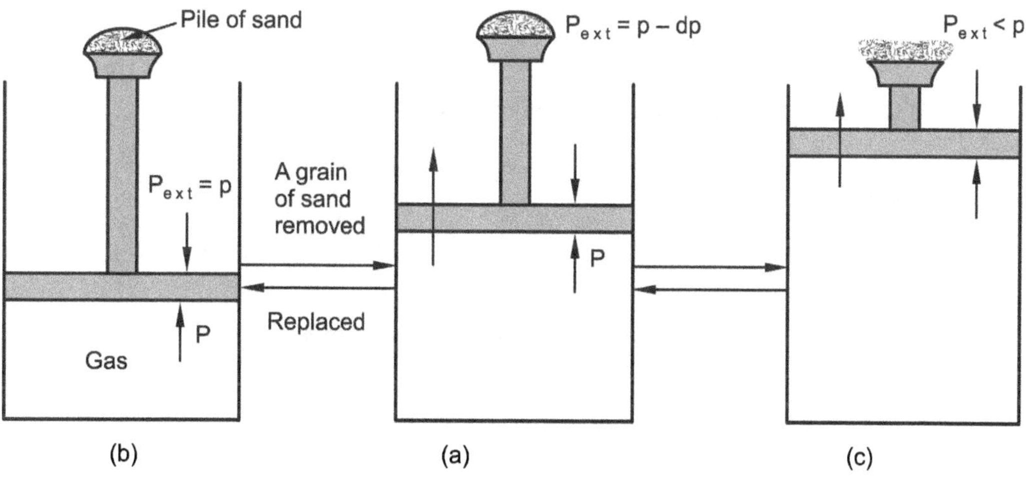

Fig. 2.4 Representation of reversible process of thermodynamics.

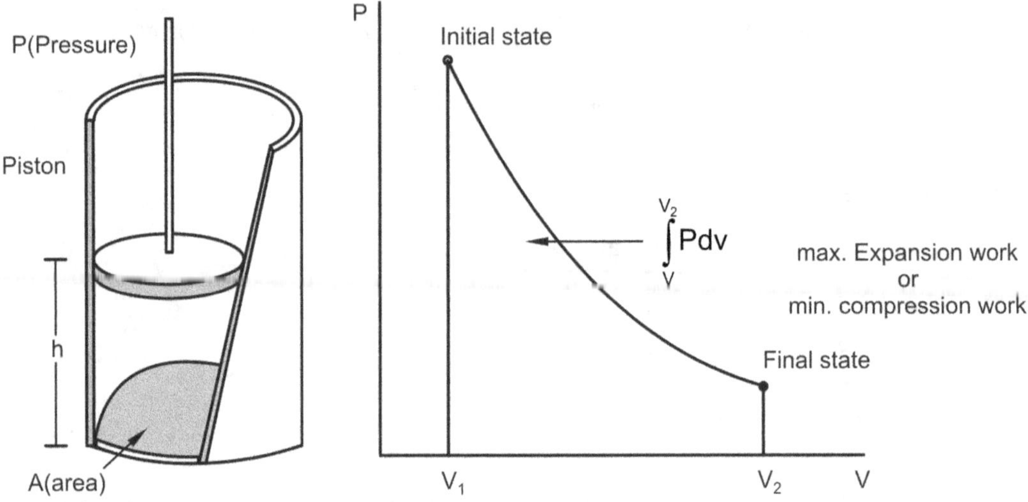

Fig. 2.5 A cylinder with a weight less and friction less piston.

The eq. (2.22) also tells about the maximum work done in the heat absorbed

We know that $\quad \Delta E = Q + W$

$$Q = \Delta E - W$$

But $\Delta E = 0$ for an ideal gas in an isothermal process.

$\therefore \quad Q = -W$

Total heat is utilized in the form of work hence maximum work is obtained.

2.4 Thermochemistry

Thermo chemistry is the study of heat changes accompanying chemical and physical processes

Heat changes measured at constant volume is represented as ΔE and that measured at constant pressure as ΔH.

i.e. $\quad Q_V = \Delta E$

$$Q_p = \Delta H$$

- During a chemical process if heat is absorbed it is said be endothermic and if it liberates it is said to be exothermic process.

$$\text{Exothermic process} = \Delta H / \Delta E = (-) \text{ value}$$

$$\text{Exothermic process} = \Delta H / \Delta E = (+) \text{ value}$$

Standard States: The usual forms of the substance (produces or reactants) either in solid, liquid or gaseous state that would ordinarily exist at 298°K or 25°C and at 1 atmp are refer to as standard states.

Ex: 1. Carbon at 25 °C exist as solid and it is taken as standard stae.

2. Oxygen exists as gas at 25 °C and it is taken as standard stae.

- The heat content of all the elements in their standard states are arbitrarily assigned values of zero.

2.4.1 Heat of Combustion

"Heat involved (liberated or absorbed) when 1 mole of a substance undergoes complete oxidation at 1 atm pressure".

Consider the reaction

$$C_{(s)} + O_{2(g)} = CO_{2(g)} \quad 94.052 \, cal$$

$$\Delta H^o_{298} = -94,052 \text{ or } 94.052 \text{ k.cal}$$

- Subscripts 's' and 'g' appearing represent solid and gas respectively.

- ΔH^o_{298} is the standard heat of reaction for the process at 298 °k or 25 °C (ΔH^o_{25})

- When pressure is not mentioned usually taken as 1 atmp.

- In the above reaction – 94.052 cal represent heat of combustion and negative sign indicate the exothermic reaction.

2.4.2 Hess Law of Heat Summation

Hess showed that in reactions ΔH depend only on the initial and final states of a system whether it involves one step (or) several steps. Therefore thermochemical equations for several steps in a reaction can be added (or) subtracted to get the heat of overall reaction. This principle is known as Hess's law of constant heat summation. It provides a means of calculating heat quantities that cannot be determined directly by experiment.

For example, the heat of combustion of carbon (graphite) to carbon monoxide is difficult to measure experimentally. However it may be obtained from the heats of combustion of carbon (graphite) to CO_2 and CO to CO_2 by subtracting as follows

$$C_{(s)} + O_{2(g)} = CO_{2(g)}; \quad \Delta H^o_{298} = -94,052 \, cal$$

$$CO_{(g)} + \frac{1}{2} O_{2(g)} = CO_{2(g)}; \quad \Delta H^o_{298} = -67,836 \, cal$$

$$\overline{C_{(s)} + \frac{1}{2} O_{2(g)} = CO_{(g)}; \quad \Delta H^o_{298} = -26,416 \, cal}$$

2.4.3 Heat of Formation

Heat of formation of a substance is the heat evolved (or) absorbed when 1 mole of a compound is formed from its constituent elements, the reactants and products being taken as in their standard states.

The heat of formation of CO_2 from its constituent elements carbon and oxygen is –94,052 cal and this is also the heat of combustion.

In calculating the heat of reaction using Hess law we can use the following equation

$$\Delta H^{\circ}_{reaction} = \Sigma H^{\circ}_{products} - \Sigma \Delta H_{reac\,tan\,ts} \qquad \qquad .....(2.24)$$

For example

The heat of formation of $CH_4 = -17,899$ Cal (ΔH°_{298})

The heat of formation of $CO_2 = -94\ 052$ Cal (ΔH°_{298})

The heat of formation of acetic acid $= -116,400$ Cal (ΔH°_{298})

Now, the heat of reaction of acetic acid from CH_4 and CO_2 is

$$CH_{4(g)} + CO_{2(g)} = CH_3COOH_{(l)}$$

Applying Hess's law

$$\Delta H^{\circ}_{298} = (-116,400\ cal) - [(-17889\ cal) + (-94,052\ cal)]$$

$$= -4459\ cal$$

The heat of formation of acetic acid from CH_4 and CO_2 is –4,459 cal and it indicates 4459 cal of heat would be liberated if 1 mole of $CH_4(g)$ and 1 mole of $CO_2(g)$ react to give 1 mole of $CH_3COOH_{(l)}$.

Heat of Solution

When a solute is dissolved in a solvent, a heat of solution is involved. This heat of solution is not generally constant for a given solute – solvent system but changes with volume of solvent used.

$\therefore$ It may be expressed as

(a) Integral heat of solution

(b) Differential heat of solution

(c) Heat of solution at infinite dilution

(a) *Integral heat of solution* is the heat effect involved when 1 mole of a solute is dissolved in a solvent to form a solution of definite concentration.

(b) *Differential heat of solution* is the heat involved when 1 mole of a solute is dissolved in a large quantities of solution of definite concentration so that no significant change in the concentration of the solution results

(c) *Heat of solution at infinite dilution* is the maximum heat of solution obtained as the volume of solvent is increased.

2.5 The Second Law of Thermodynamics

The first law only tells us about the conservation of energy and its conversion from one form to another form but it says nothing about the probability of the reaction whether it will occur or not.

But the second law refers to the probability of occurrence of a process based on the tendency of the system to approach a state of energy equilibrium.

In general most of the natural phenomenons occur spontaneously in one direction.

For example

Heat flows from hotter to colder bodies spontaneously. Gases expand from higher pressure to lower pressure region.

Solute molecules diffuse from region of higher concentration to lower concentration region.

These spontaneous processes will not occur in a reverse manner until some external force is applied.

Now, the second law can be stated as:

"A steam engine can do work only with a fall in temperature and a flow of heat to the lower temperature. No useful work can be obtained from heat at constant temperature".

The spontaneous character of natural processes and the limitations on the conversion of heat into work is explained by the second law.

The Efficiency of a Heat Engine

Efficiency of a steam engine is nothing but how much of the heat energy that is available is converted into useful work and we should remember that all the heat available can never be converted into work completely.

Suppose let us consider a steam engine having two heat reservoirs one is source and other sink, at two different temperatures. At source heat is absorbed and only a part is converted into useful work (w) and remaining is transmitted to the sink.

The fraction of heat that is converted into work is taken as 'Q', and then efficiency of engine is

$$\text{Efficiency} = \frac{W}{Q} \qquad \qquad .....(2.25)$$

We should remember that even the efficiency of even hypothetical heat engine operating without friction can be unity or 100% because 'W' is always less than Q in conversion of heat to work.

Imagine a hypothetical steam engine operating reversibly at two different temperature T_{hot} (upper temperature) and T_{cold} (lower temperature).

It absorbs Q_{hot} from the source and in it some amount is converted into work 'w' in the form of steam, than returns the remaining amount Q_{cold} to the cold reservoir (or) sink present at a temperature of T_{cold}.

Now to find the efficiency of such systems carnot gave the following equation

$$\frac{W}{Q_{hot}} = \frac{Q_{hot} - Q_{cold}}{Q_{hot}} \qquad \qquad .....(2.26)$$

But heat flow (Q) proportional to temperature gradient

$$\frac{Q_{hot}}{Q_{cold}} = \frac{T_{hot}}{T_{cold}} \qquad \qquad .....(2.27)$$

By combining these two eqs. (26, 27) we can determine efficiency

$$\text{Efficiency} = \frac{Q_{hot} - Q_{cold}}{Q_{hot}} = \frac{T_{hot} - T_{cold}}{T_{hot}} \qquad \qquad .....(2.28)$$

Key points

(i)   As the T_{hot} becomes higher, efficiency of the engine increases,

(ii)   When the T_{cold} becomes absolute zero on Kelvin scale the 'E' is unity (But never possible).

(iii)   If $T_{hot} = T_{cold}$ the cycle is isothermal and efficiency is zero.

2.5.1 Concept of Entropy

For a reversible carnot cycle operating between temperature T_2 and T_1 we know that (from eq 2.28).

$$\frac{Q_2 - Q_1}{Q_2} = \frac{T_2 - T_1}{T_2} \qquad \qquad .....(i)$$

where Q_2 is the heat absorbed isothermally and reversibly at temperature T_2

Q_1 is the heat lost isothermally and reversibly at temperature T_1

Rearranging the above eq. (i)

$$1 - \frac{Q_2}{Q_1} = 1 - \frac{T_2}{T_1}$$

$$\Rightarrow \frac{Q_2}{T_2} = \frac{Q_1}{T_1} \qquad \qquad \dots\dots(ii)$$

Thus in general $\qquad \dfrac{Q}{T} = \text{constant} \qquad \qquad \dots\dots(2.29)$

From this it is evident that heat absorbed or lost isothermally divided by the temperature at which heat is absorbed or lost is a constant quantity for a particular system:

In the equation (ii) $\qquad Q_2$ is heat absorbed at T_2

Q_1 is heat lost at T_1

By taking the sings (+) for heat absorbed and (–) for heat evolved eq. (ii) can be written as

$$\frac{Q_2}{T_2} = \frac{-Q_1}{T_1}$$

$$\frac{Q_2}{T_2} + \frac{Q_1}{T_1} = 0 \qquad \qquad \dots\dots(2.30)$$

Thus we can say that when the isothermal and adiabatic processes in a carnot cycle are carried out reversibly, the summation of $\dfrac{Q}{T}$ is equal to zero

$$\Sigma \frac{Q}{T} = 0 \qquad \qquad \dots\dots(2.31)$$

Thus, Carnot recognised that when Q_{rev}, a path dependant property is divided by T a new path-independent properly is generated called "Entropy" it is defined as

$$\Delta S = \frac{Q_{rev}}{T} \qquad \qquad \dots\dots(2.32)$$

Entropy Change in Reversible Process

Consider a process occurring under completely reversible conditions i.e. the heat is absorbed and lost by the surroundings reversibly. If Q_{rev} is the heat absorbed by the system then Q_{rev} will be lost by surroundings.

Now, if this process takes place isothermally at absolute temperature 'T' then:

(I) Entropy change in the system $= \dfrac{Q_{rev}}{T} \left(\Delta S_{system} - \dfrac{Q_{rev}}{T} \right)$

(ii) Entropy change in the surroundings $\Delta S_{surroundies} = \dfrac{-Q_{rev}}{T}$

Then total entropy change

$$\Delta S_{system} + \Delta S_{surrounds} = \dfrac{Q_{rev}}{T} + \left(-\dfrac{Q_{rev}}{T} \right)$$

$$= \dfrac{Q_{rev}}{T} - \dfrac{Q_{rev}}{T}$$

$$= 0$$

Thus in a "reversible process" net Entropy change for a combined system and surroundings is zero i.e. in a thermodynamically reversible process, the Entropy of the system and its surroundings remains unaltered

$$\Delta S_{universe} = \Delta S_{system} + \Delta S_{surr} = 0 \qquad \qquad ......(2.33)$$

But in the case of irreversible (spontaneous process) the entropy change of the total system (or) universe is always positive because ΔS_{surr} is always less than DS_{syst} in an irreversible process

Thus $\qquad\qquad \Delta S_{universe} = \Delta S_{system} + \Delta S_{sor} > 0 \qquad\qquad .....(2.34)$

This can serve as a criterion of spontaneity of a real process.

Thus according to one of the definitions of the second law all spontaneous processes are thermodynamically irreversible. We can say that "all spontaneous processes are accompanied by a net increase of entropy".

In a reversible process, the entropy of the system and the surroundings taken together remains constant while in an irreversible process the entropy of the system and the surroundings increases.

Physical Significance of Entropy

Entropy is regarded as a measure of the disorder or randomness of a system. More the disorderness more is the entropy.

All spontaneous processes like diffusion of gases, heat flow etc. lead to a state of more randomness i.e. every spontaneous process leads to an increase in entropy.

Consider a molecular system in states A and B as shown in Fig. 2.6. In state A all the molecules are arranged in orderly manner, while in state B the molecules are present at random and it is highly disordered.

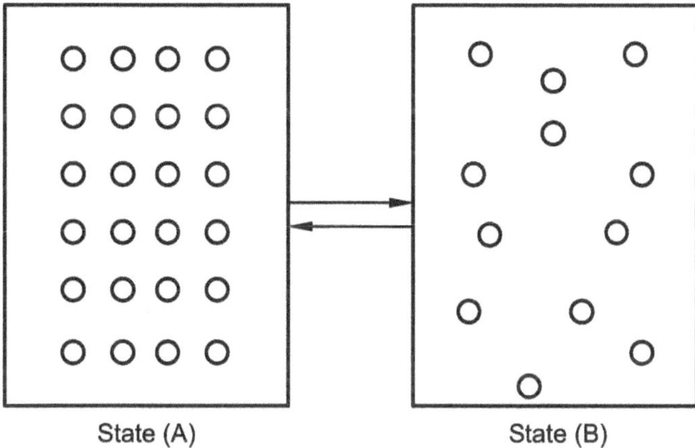

Fig. 2.6 States of Molecular systems

- In state A since all the molecules are in orderly manner it has less entropy while in state B due to more randomness it has more entropy,

Thus

Any change in a system which is accompanied by an increase in entropy tends to be spontaneous.

(i) Entropy change in the system $= \dfrac{Q_{rev}}{T}\left(\Delta S_{system} = \dfrac{Q_{rev}}{T}\right)$

(ii) Entropy change in the surroundings $\Delta S_{surroundies} = \dfrac{-Q_{rev}}{T}$

Then total entropy change

$$\Delta S_{system} + \Delta S_{sorrads} = \dfrac{Q_{rev}}{T} + \left(\dfrac{-Q_{rev}}{T}\right)$$

$$= \dfrac{Q_{rev}}{T} - \dfrac{Q_{rev}}{T}$$

$$= 0$$

Entropy Change Accompanying Phase Change

When even phase conversion takes place either from solid to liquid, liquid to gas (or) vice versa the temperature, pressure remains constant and it is called latent heat.

The Entropy change for such process can be calculated by

$$\Delta S_m = \frac{\Delta H_m}{T_m} \qquad \text{(Entropy change of melting)} \qquad .....(2.35)$$

$$\Delta S_v = \frac{\Delta H_v}{T_b} \qquad \text{(Entropy change of evaporation)} \qquad .....(2.36)$$

where

ΔH_m = Latent heat of melting for 1 mole

T_m = Melting temperature

ΔH_v = Latent heat of vaporisation for 1 mole

T_b = Boiling temperature

Note: eq. (2.32) can be written in the form of heat capacities as

$$\frac{dq_{rev}}{T} = \frac{C_p dT}{T} = dS$$

(Heat absorbed at constant pressure ($dq_p = C_p dT$) for reversible process) = eq. (2.32(a)

2.6 The Third Law of Thermodynamics

This law states that the Entropy (disorderness) of a pure crystalline substance is zero at absolute zero because the crystal arrangement should show greater orderliness at that temperature, but attaining that temperature is impossible even with sophisticated process also. This law helps in calculating the entropy of pure substances by the equation.

$$S_T = \Sigma \frac{dq_{rev}}{T_i} + S_0 \qquad .....(2.37)$$

where

S_0 = Molar entropy at absolute zero

S_T = absolute molar entropy at any temperature

This equation is a rearranged eq. 32-a. When magnitude dq_{rev} is replaced by the terms CpdT at constant pressure, thus making it possible to determine entropy by knowing heat capacities and entropy change during a phase change as the temperature raises from O K to T.

From the following equation 'S_T' for a substance that undergoes two phase changes melting (m) and vapourization (V) can be determined as

$$S_T = \int_0^{T_m} \frac{C_p dT}{T} + \frac{\Delta H_m}{T_m} + \int_{T_m}^{T_v} \frac{C_p dT}{T} + \frac{\Delta H_v}{T_v} + \int_{T_v}^{T} \frac{C_p dT}{T} \quad .....(2.38)$$

Key points

- Since $S_0 = 0$ it has to be omitted

- Each of these terms can be evaluated independently, the first integral is calculated by plotting C_p/T vs T.

- $Dq_{rev} = C_p dT$ [used in reversible systems]

- So replaced by $\left(\dfrac{\Delta H_r}{T} \right)$

2.6.1 Helmholtz Free Energy or Work Function

The total internal energy of a system is a combination of isothermally available internal energy for doing work (A) and isothermally unavailable internal energy (TS) for doing work

i.e. $\quad\quad\quad\quad E = A + TS$ $\quad\quad\quad\quad\quad\quad\quad .....(2.39)$

This equation can be written for Helmholtz free energy which is defined as the internal energy minus isothermally unavailable internal energy

$\quad\quad\quad\quad A = E - TS$ $\quad\quad\quad\quad\quad\quad\quad .....(2.40)$

where A = Helmholtz free energy

Now, consider a system undergoing any physical or chemical process, then the driving force to that is 'A' (a part of internal energy), which can be proved as follow.

Since the system is undergoing change

$\quad\quad\quad\quad \Delta A = \Delta E - \Delta(TS)$ $\quad\quad\quad\quad\quad\quad .....(2.41)$

At constant temperature

$\quad\quad\quad\quad \Delta A = \Delta E - T\Delta S$ $\quad\quad\quad\quad\quad\quad .....(2.42)$

But $(\Delta E = Q - W)$

$\therefore \quad\quad\quad\quad \Delta A = Q - W - T\Delta S$ $\quad\quad\quad\quad\quad .....(2.43)$

From definition of entropy $\Delta S = \dfrac{Q_{rev}}{T}$

$$Q_{rev} = T\Delta S$$

Substituting the value in eq. (2.43)

$$\Delta A = T\Delta S - W_{max} - T\Delta S$$

$$\Delta A = -W_{max} \qquad\qquad .....(2.44)$$

or $\qquad\qquad -\Delta A = W_{max}$

Thus Helmholtz free energy (A) is the energy available to do PV work in a reversible isothermal process.

2.6.2 Gibb's Free Energy

It is nothing but the isothermally available energy at constant temperature and pressure.

It is equal to total heat minus isothermally unavailable energy

$$G = H - TS \qquad\qquad .....(2.45)$$

The following differential forms of equations are useful in the study of reversible processes.

$\Rightarrow \qquad\qquad G = H - TS \qquad$ (But $H = E + PV$)

$\Rightarrow \qquad\qquad G = E + PV - TS \qquad\qquad .....(2.46)$

on partial differentiation of above equation

$$dG = dE + PdV + Vdp - Tds - SdT \qquad\qquad .....(2.47)$$

$$\text{But} \begin{cases} dE = q_{rev} - Pdv \text{ (First law)} \\ q_{rev} = Tds \end{cases}$$

$\Rightarrow$ So, $\qquad dG = q_{rev} - PdV + pdV + Vdp - Tds - SdT \qquad .....(2.48)$

$\qquad\qquad dG = Tds - PdV + PdV + Vdp - Tds - SdT \qquad .....(2.49)$

on simplify $\qquad dG = Vdp - SdT \qquad\qquad .....(2.50)$

At constant pressure $Vdp = 0$

$\therefore \qquad\qquad dG = -SdT \text{ or } \left(\dfrac{\partial G}{\partial T}\right)_p = -S \qquad\qquad .....(2.51)$

At constant temperature $SdT = 0$

$$dG = Vdp \text{ or } \left(\dfrac{\partial G}{\partial T}\right)_T = V \qquad\qquad .....(2.52)$$

But from ideal 995 $\quad V = \dfrac{nRT}{V}$

$\therefore \qquad \left(\dfrac{\partial G}{\partial P}\right)_T = \dfrac{nRT}{P}$ .....(2.53)

or $\qquad \partial G = nRT \dfrac{\partial p}{p}$ .....(2.54)

This on integration between G_2 at P_2 and G_1 at P_1

$$\left(G_2 - G_1\right) = \Delta G = nRT \, ln \dfrac{P_2}{P_1}$$ .....(2.55)

Apply log $\qquad \Delta G = 2.303 \, nRT \, \log \dfrac{P_2}{P_1}$ .....(2.56)

where ΔG is the free energy change of an ideal gas undergoing an isothermal reversible or irreversible process.

2.6.3 Clausius – Clapeyron Equation

Consider a beaker containing water in liquid and vapour state which are in equilibrium with each other and the molar free energy changes of these are equal.

$$dG_l = dG_v$$ .....(2.57)

In phase change the free energy change for 1 mole of liquid vapour is

$$dG_v = Vdp - SdT$$ .....(2.58)

$\therefore \qquad$ From

$\Rightarrow \qquad V_1 dp - S_1 dT = V_v dp - S_v dT$ .....(2.59)

$\Rightarrow \qquad \dfrac{dp}{dT} = \dfrac{S_v - S_l}{V_v - V_l} = \dfrac{\Delta S}{\Delta V}$ .....(2.60)

But at constant pressure, heat absorbed in reversible process is equal to the molar heat of vapourization and from second law

$$\Delta S = \dfrac{\Delta H_v}{T}$$ .....(2.61)

Substitute this equation into eq. 2.60

$$\frac{dp}{dT} = \frac{\Delta H_v}{T\Delta V} \qquad\qquad .....(2.62)$$

(Where $DV = V_v - V_l$)

This equation is known as clapeyron equation

We know that the vapour will obey the ideal gas law

$$PV = nRT \quad (n = 1)$$

$$V_v = \frac{RT}{P} \quad (V = V_v)$$

Further V_l is insignificant compared to V_v hence it can be neglected. By substituting these in to eq. (2.60) we get

$$= \frac{dp}{dT} = \frac{\Delta S}{V_v - 0} \Rightarrow \frac{dp}{dT} = \frac{\Delta S}{V_v} \qquad\qquad .....(2.63)$$

$$= \frac{dp}{dT} = \frac{\Delta S}{RT/p} \Rightarrow \frac{dp}{dT} = \frac{P.\Delta S}{RT} \quad \text{But } \Delta S = \frac{\Delta H_v}{T}$$

$$= \frac{dp}{dT} = \frac{p.\Delta HV}{RT^2} \qquad\qquad .....(2.64)$$

This is known as Clausius – Clapeyron equation.

Now Assuming ΔH_v as constant and integrating between limits of the vapour pressure P_1 and P_2 to corresponding temperatures T_1 and T_2 we get

$$\int_{P_1}^{P_2} \frac{dp}{p} = \frac{\Delta H}{R} \int_{T_1}^{T_2} T^{-2} dT \qquad\qquad .....(2.65)$$

$$\left[\ln p\right]_{P_1}^{P_2} = \frac{\Delta H_v}{R}\left[\left(-\frac{1}{T_2} - \left(-\frac{1}{T_1}\right)\right)\right] \qquad\qquad .....(2.66)$$

$$\ln P_2 - \ln P_1 = \frac{\Delta H_v}{R}\left[\frac{1}{T_1} - \frac{1}{T_2}\right] \qquad\qquad .....(2.67)$$

Finally
$$\frac{ln\,P_2}{P_1} = \frac{\Delta H_v (T_2 - T_1)}{RT_1 T_2} = 0 \qquad \ldots\ldots(2.68)$$

or
$$\log\frac{P_2}{P_1} = \frac{\Delta H_v (T_2 - T_1)}{2.303 RT_1 T_2} = 0 \qquad \ldots\ldots(2.69)$$

This equation is used to calculate the mean heat of vaporization of a liquid if its vapour pressure at two temperature is available.

- If suppose if the mean heat of vapourization and the vapour pressure at one temperature are known the vapour pressure at another temperature can be obtained.

- The Clapeyron and Clasius – Clapeyron equations are important in the study of various phase transitions and in the development of the equations of some colligative properties.

2.6.4 The Van't Hoff Equation

The effect of temperature on equilibrium constants is obtained by writing the equation

$$ln\,k = \frac{\Delta G^\circ}{RT} \qquad \ldots\ldots(2.70)$$

Now, differentiating it with respect to temperature

$$\frac{d\,ln\,k}{dT} = \frac{-1}{R}\frac{d\left(\Delta G^\circ / T\right)}{dT} \qquad \ldots\ldots(2.71)$$

The Gibbs – Helmholtz equation can be written in the form of

$$\frac{d\left(\Delta G / T\right)}{dT} = \frac{-\Delta H}{T^2} \qquad \ldots\ldots(2.72)$$

Now substituting the eq. (2.72) into eq. (2.71) we get

$$\frac{d\,ln\,k}{dT} = \frac{\Delta H^\circ}{RT^2} \qquad \ldots\ldots(2.73)$$

where ΔH° = Standard Enthalpy of reaction

The eq. (2.73) is known as Van't Hoff equation

Now taking DH° as constant over the temperature range considered it becomes

$$ln\ \frac{k_2}{k_1} = \frac{\Delta H°}{R}\left(\frac{T_2 - T_1}{T_1 T_2}\right) \qquad .....(2.74)$$

- This eq. (2.74) helps to calculate the Enthalpy reaction if the equilibrium constants at T_1 and T_2 are known

- DH° varies with temperature.

- The solubility of a solid in an ideal solution is a special type of equilibrium and solubility can be written as

$$ln\ \frac{X_2}{X_1} = \frac{\Delta H_f}{R}\left(\frac{T_2 - T_1}{T_1 T_2}\right) \qquad .....(2.75)$$

2.7 Questions

1. Distinguish between reversible and irreversible process.

2. State and explain first law of thermodynamics. How does the equation take different forms under different thermodynamic situations.

3. What is an entropy. How do you predict the spontaneity of a process using the concept of entropy.

4. State the third law of thermodynamics and derive "Gibb's Free Energy" equation.

CHAPTER 3

PHYSICAL PROPERTIES OF DRUG MOLECULES

3.1 Introduction

A study of physical properties of drug molecules is a important for product formulation. We can understand the relationship between a drugs's molecular and physiochemical properties and its structure and action. These properties come from molecular bonding order of atoms in a molecule. They may be either additive or constitute properties.

Additive properties: Derived from sum of the properties individual atoms or functional groups with in the molecule. E.g., mass is an additive property.

Constitutive properties: Dependent on the structural arrangement of the atoms within the molecule. E.g., Optical rotation (Depends on chirality of molecules, determined by atomic bonding order).

- Many physical properties are constitutive yet have some measures of additive.

- Physical properties encompass the specific relations between the atoms in molecules and well-defined forms of energy or other external "Yard sticks" of measurement. *E.g.,* The concept of weight uses the force of gravity as an external measure to compare the mass of objects, where as that of optical rotation uses plane-polarised light to describe the optical rotation of molecules organized in a particular bonding pattern.

By carefully associating specific physical properties with the chemical nature of closely related molecules one can:

(a)   provide evidence for relative chemical (or) physical behaviour of a molecule.

(b)   Describe the spatial arrangement of atoms in drug molecule.

(c)   Suggest methods for the qualitative and quantitative analysis of a particular pharmaceutical agent.

a, b describes about the chemical nature and potential action necessary for creation of new molecules with selective pharmacological activity.

C provides the researcher with tools for drug design and manufacturing and offers the analyst a wide range of methods for assessing the quality of drug products.

Physical properties of molecules have expanded greatly and with increasing advances computer-based computational tools to develop molecules with ideal physical properties has the great impact of computational modelling. The computational tools offer great promise for enhancing the speed of drug design and selection

E.g., Computer modelling of therapeutic targets.

(E.g., HIV protease) based on screening of known or predicted physical properties.

- Computational programs can then be utilized to computer the no. of molecules that make reasonable drugs based on these molecular restrictions.

- Finally, the ability to measure the physical properties of lead compound is critical to assuring that during the transition from computer to large-scale manufacturing, the initially identified molecules remains physically the same. This is a guideline that the Food and Drug Administration (FDA) required to ensure human safety and drug efficacy.

3.2 Dielectric Constant

- Dielectric constant is represented by the symbol 'ε'
- Dielectric constant ordinarily has no dimensions because it is the ratio of two capacitances.
- It has no units.
- Dielectric constant of vacuum is unity.

To properly discuss dipoles and the effects of solvation, one must understand the concepts of polarity and dielectric constant. Placing molecules in an electric field is one way to induce a dipole.

Consider two parallel conducting plates, such as plates of electric condenser, separated by some medium across a distance r, and apply a potential across the plates. Electricity will flow from left plate to right plate through the battery until the potential difference of plates equals to battery supplying the initial potential difference.

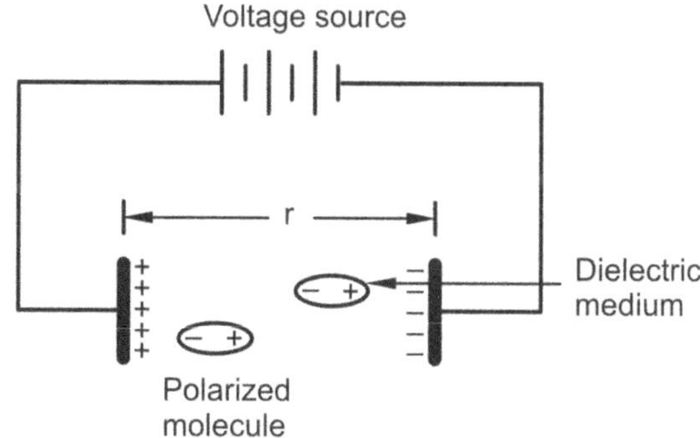

Fig. 3.1 Parallel plate condenser

The capacitance (C, in farads [F]) is equal to the quantity of electric charge (q. in coulombs) stored on the plates divided by the potential difference (V, in volts) between the plates:

$$C = q/V$$

Capacitance of the condenser depends on the type of medium separating the plates as well as on the thickness r. When a vacuum fills the space between the plates, the capacitance is C_0. This value is used as a reference to compare capacitances when other substances fill the space. If H_2O fills the space, the capacitance is increased because the water molecule can orientate itself so that its negative end lies nearest the positive condenser plate and its positive end lies nearest the negative plate. Electrons can flow between the plates. Additional charge can be placed on the plates per unit of applied voltage.

The capacitance of condenser filled with some material C_x, divided by the reference standard. C_0, is referred to as the dielectric constant, ε:

$$\varepsilon = \frac{C_x}{C_0} = \frac{\text{Capacitance of condenser with liquid}}{\text{Capacitance of conderser in vaccum}}$$

The liquid whose dielectric constant is being measured is kept in container between the two plates and measured.

Dielectric constant of a substance is a measure of efficiency to induce dipoles in another molecule. It is a physiochemical property.

Applications

1. *Polarity scales:* Dielectric constant is widely used for measuring in g polarity of solvents. As per values of dielectric constants, solvents can be arranged in the form of scale. The scale is with (1) for vacuum at one end, 78.5 for H_2O at other end. This scale is used to select a solvent with appropriate polarity.

2. *Solubilization of drugs:* Drugs are either non-polar or semipolar. When and non-polar molecule is added to water, dipolar water molecules induce a partial charge on the non-polar molecules by attracting and repelling the electrons. Uneven electronic distribution of electrons leads to induced dipoles. The higher the magnitude of the dielectric constant, the greater the solvation energy of the solvent, hence greater is the solubility. This is used for preparation of solutions for liquid orals and injections.

   E.g., Bartbiturates and Xanthine derivatives dielectric constant is reported.

3.3 Dielectric Constant of Solvent

Selection of a Solvent for the Solubility of Drugs

Dielectric requirement is defined as the dielectric constant of solvent blend at which the solubility of solute is maximum.

The dielectric constant for a blend can be calculated using equation.

$$\text{Dielectric constant of solvent bend} = \frac{\%\,\text{solvent A} \times \varepsilon \,\text{of A} + \%\,\text{solvent B} \times \varepsilon \,\text{of B}}{100}$$

E.g., dielectric constants of ethanol and water are 24.3 and 78.5 respectively.

A solvent blend is prepared by mixing 90:10 ethanol-water.

$$\text{The dielectric constant of blend} = \frac{[(90 \times 24.3) + (10 \times 78.5)]}{100}$$

$$= 29.7$$

If non-polar molecules in suitable solvents are placed between the plates of a charged capacitor, an induced polarization of the molecules occur, the induced polarization occurs because when the electric charges are separated in between the parallel plates when they are in electric field. The electrons and nuclei are also displaced from their original position in this induction process. This temporary induced dipole moment is proportional to the strength of capacitor and induced polarizability (α_p).

This temporary induced dipole moment is proportional to the field strength of capacitor and the induced polarizability, α p, which is a characteristic property of the particular molecule.

Polarizability is defined as the ease with which an ion molecule can be polarised by any external force like selective field, electric light energy or another molecule.

From electromagnetic theory, it is possible to obtain the relationship

$$\frac{\varepsilon-1}{\varepsilon+2}=\frac{4}{3}\pi n \propto p$$

n is the no. of molecules per unit volume.

Equation is known as Clausius-Mossoti equation.

Multiply both sides by the molecular weight of substance, M, and dividing both sides by the solvent density, ρ

$$\left(\frac{\varepsilon-1}{\varepsilon+2}\right)\frac{M}{\rho}=\frac{4}{3}\frac{\pi n M \propto p}{P}=\frac{4}{3}\pi N \propto p = pi$$

N is Avogadro's number, 6.023×10^{23} mole^{-1}.

Pi is induced molar polarization

Pi represents the induced dipole moment per mole of non-polar substance. When the electric field strength of condenser, v/m in volts per meter, is unity.

When non-polar molecules like pentane are placed in a suitable solvent between the plates of a charged capacitor, an induced polarization of the molecules can occur. Again, this induced dipole occurs because of the separation of electric charge with the molecule due to the electric field generated between the plates.

3.4 Dipole Moment

Dipole moment is represented by the symbol (μ) units of dipole moment are debye:

$$1 \text{debye} = 10^{-18} \text{ e.s.u (electro static unit)}$$

In S.I units $\qquad$ 1 debye = 3.3×10^{-30} columbs.

In a polar molecule, the separation of positively and negatively charged regions can be permanent, and the molecule will possess a permanent dipole 'μ.'

Perfect arrangement of molecules contains maximum dipole moment. Many of molecules may not have maximum dipole moment because of improper alignment of charges.

Dipolar molecule is defined as the one in which the regions of positive and negative changes are well separated due to uneven distribution of electrons in the molecule.

Definition: It is defined as the vector equal in magnitude to the product of electric charge and distance, having the direction of the line joining the positive and negative centres.

$$\text{Dipole moment} = \text{distance} \times \text{charge}$$

$$\mu = r \times e$$

S.I units:	c.m	metre	coulombs

C.G.S system   unit is debye

$$p = p_i + p_o = \left(\frac{E-1}{E+2} \right) \frac{H}{p}$$

P_o is orientation polarization of permanent dipoles

where $\qquad p_o = \dfrac{4\pi N\mu^2}{9KT}$

N = Avagadro number

μ = dipole moment

K = Boltzmann constant $(1.38 \times 10^{-23} \text{ JK}^{-1})$

T = temperature

Since $\qquad p_o$ depends on temperature

$$p = p_i + A. \frac{1}{T}$$

If graph is plotted against the pressure and temperature $\left(\dfrac{1}{T} \right)$ the slope of graph can be used to calculate μ.,where p_i is y-intercept. Value of p can be obtained by measuring dielectric constant and density of polar compound at various temperatures.

$$\text{Slope A is } \frac{4\pi N\mu^2}{9K}.$$

E.g: Dipolar molecules are water, HCl etc. In water, oxygen is an electronegative atom that has a greater tendency to draw the shared pair of electrons towards it. Hydrogen atom assumes the charge as the shared electron pair is away from it. Thus +ve and –ve centres are developed in a molecule.

Some solutes are symmetric planer. Their dipole moments are zero. Ion-induced dipole interactions are also responsible for solubility.

Applications

1. ***Crystalline nature of solids:*** If solids are dipolar molecules, the dipole moment contributes to orientation of molecules in solution.

   e.g., Ice crystals are organised through their dipole forces.

2. ***Drug-receptor interaction:*** Dipole forces are responsible for the inter action of drugs with receptors.

3. ***Therapeutic activity of drugs:*** Permanent dipole moment can be correlated with the biological activity. E.g., Insecticidal activity of DDT correlated with the structural requirements.

   DDT is available in three isomers. The activities and their dipole moments are given

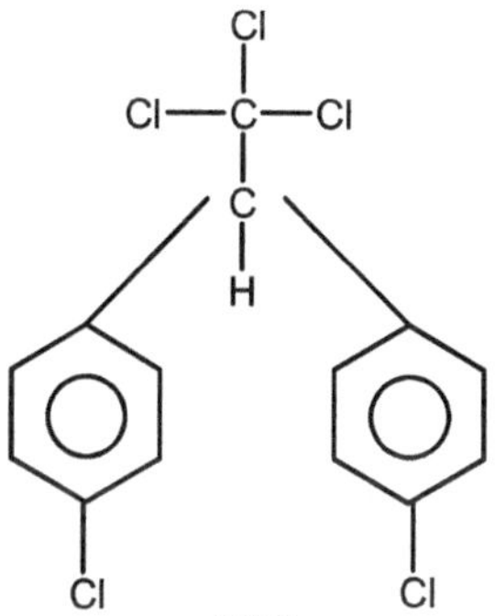

DDT
Para isomer
μ = 1.10 d
less water soluble
more lipid soluble
more toxic

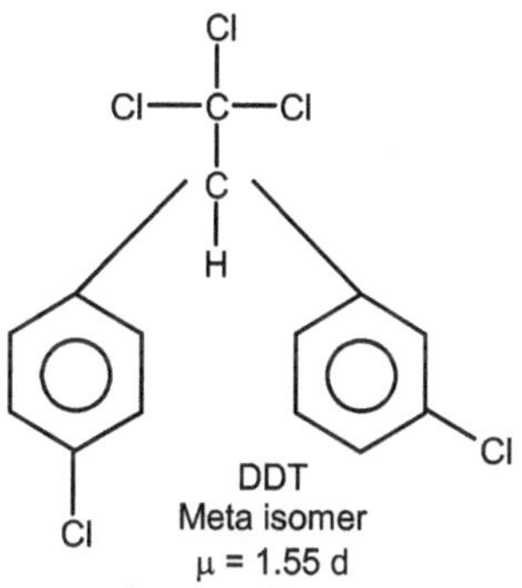

DDT
Meta isomer
μ = 1.55 d
Intermediate water
soluble intermediate
lipid soluble
intermediate toxicity

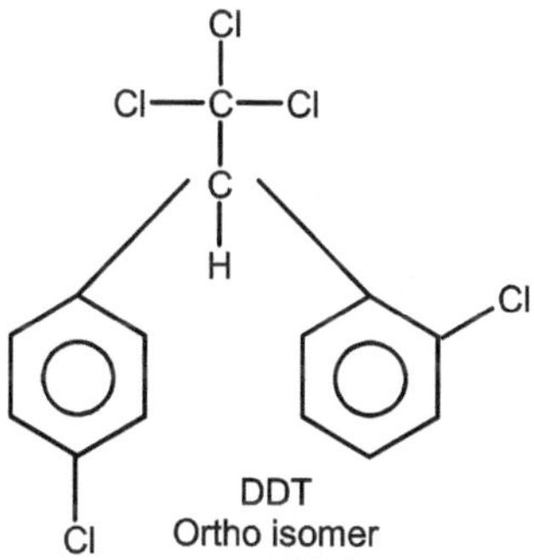

DDT
Ortho isomer
μ = 1.90 d
More water
soluble less
lipid soluble
least toxic

Refractive Index and Molar Refraction

Refractive under is represented by the symbol $[n]_D^{20}$

As it is a ratio it has no units.

Definition: It is defined as the ratio of angle of incidence to the angle of refraction.

$$\eta = \frac{\sin i}{\sin r}$$

$$\eta = \frac{\text{Velocity of light in vaccum (or) air}}{\text{Velocity of light in liquid}} = \frac{C_1}{C_2}$$

where $\sin i$ = sin of angle of incident ray of light

         $\sin r$ = sine of angle of refracted ray

         C_1 and C_2 are speeds of light.

The refractive index, by this convention, is greater than 1 for substances denser than air. Theoretically, the reference state where n = 1 should be for light passing through a vacuum; the use of air as a reference produces a differences in n of only 0.03% from the vacuum and is more commonly used.

The refractive index varies with the wave length of light and the temperature because both alter the energy of interaction.

E.g., n_D^{20} signifies the refractive index using the D-line emission of sodium, at 589 nm, at a temperature of 20 °C. Pressure must also be held constant in measuring the refractive index of gases.

The refractive index can be used to

1. Identify a substance

2. To measure its purity

3. To determine the concentration of one substance dissolved in another.

Refractometers are used to determine refractive index. These play important role in studying pharmaceutical compounds that do not under go extensive UV-v is absorption due to their electronic structure.

The equations

$$\left(\frac{\varepsilon - 1}{\varepsilon + 2}\right) = \frac{4}{3}\pi n \propto p$$

Polarizability can be made a molecular property i.e., molar polarizability, by multiplying both sides by molecular mass of the substance (M) and dividing by density

(ρ). The equation:

$$\frac{(\varepsilon-1)M}{(\varepsilon+2)\rho} = \frac{4\pi n\alpha_p M}{3\rho} = \frac{4}{3}\pi N\alpha_p$$

N = Avogadro's number

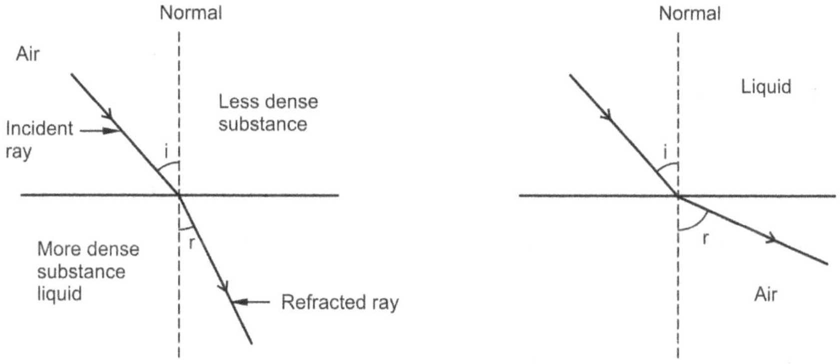

(a) Light passing less dense
to denser medium

(b) Light passing from denser
to less dense medium

Fig. 3.2 Refraction of light.

Para isomer of DDT is highly toxic and it has the least dipole moment. Lower the dipole moment, lower is its solubility in water. Para isomers have greater solubility in non-polar solvents.

E.g., Membranes of insects are lipoidal in nature, the p-isomers being soluble in non-polar solvents, can easily penetrate through the lipoidal membranes of insects.

The other isomers penetrate through the membrane at a slow rate due to their high dipole moment.

Therefore they produce less toxicity to the insects.

Chemical Structure of Compounds

   (i)   Deciding ionic nature of a bond
   (ii)   Identifying the shape of molecules
   (iii) Identifying the shape and bond angle
   (iv)   Deciding the arrangement of groups
   (v)   Identifying geometric isomers.

3.5 Induced Polarizability- Induced Dipole Moment

Induced polarizability is a characteristic of a molecule.

Polarizability: It is defined as the ease with which an ion or molecule can be polarized by an external force.

In the influence of electric field, dipoles can also have induced dipoles which facilitate further alignment of negatively charged centres closer to positively charged centres. $\because$ chlorine molecule (Cl_2) gets polarised and develops charges. This is called induced dipole moment.

Maximum dipole moment occurs when the molecules are oriented in a perfect manner.

Clausius-Mosotti equation expresses the relationship between induced polarizability of a molecule and dielectric constant. The equation

$$\frac{(\varepsilon-1)}{(\varepsilon+2)}=\frac{4}{3}\pi n \propto p$$

n = no. of molecules per unit volume

α_p = induced polarizability, m^3/mol

ε = dielectric constant.

The total molar polarization p, is the sum of induction and permanent dipole effects.

$$p = p_i + p_o = \left(\frac{\varepsilon-1}{\varepsilon+2}\right)\frac{M}{\rho}$$

p_o is the orientation polarization of permanent dipoles

$$p_o = \frac{4\pi N\mu^2}{9KT}$$

p = polarization due to orientation of permanent dipoles.

p_i = y-intercept

If p is obtained at several temperatures and plotted against $\frac{1}{T}$. The slope of the graph can be used to calculate μ and the intercept can be applied to compute α_p.

For ionic solutes and non-polar solvents ion induced dipole interaction has an essential role in solubility phenomena. For drug-receptor binding, dipole-dipole interactions are having an essential non covalent forces that contribute to enhance the pharmacologic effect. For instance, water molecules in ice crystals are organized through their dipole forces.

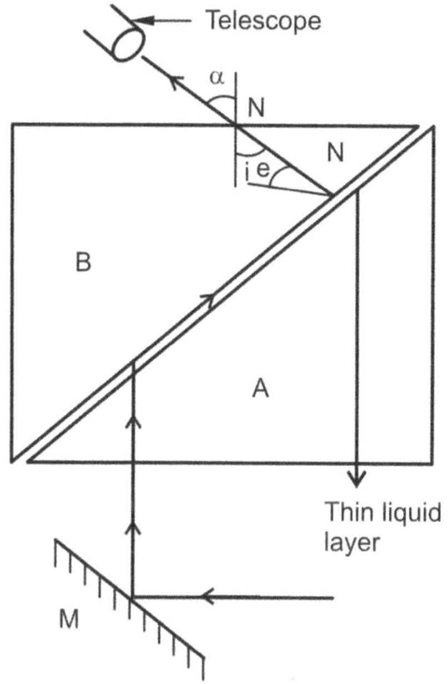

(a) Optical system showing
   the course of light ray

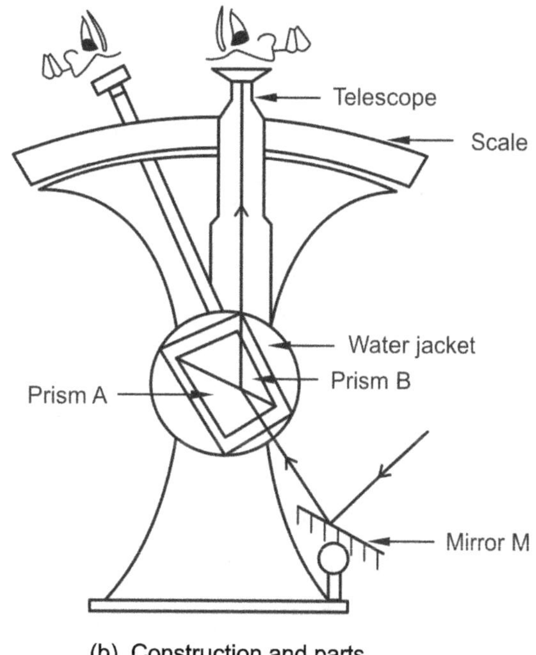

(b) Construction and parts

Fig. 3.3

3.6 Optical Rotation

- Optical rotation is represented by the symbol $[\alpha]_D^{25}$

- Optical activity is the ability of certain substances to rotate the plane of plane-polarised light.

- Optically active substances are the substances which can rotate the plane of plane-polarised light either to right-side or to left-side.

When viewed through the path of beam, if the rotation of plane polarised light takes place in clock-wise direction, it is called as dextrorotary. If the rotation of plane-polarised light takes place in anticlockwise direction (left), then the rotation is called levorotatory. Optical rotation is prefixed with the symbols, (+) for dextro rotation, (−) for levorotation.

Optical rotation α, depends on the density of the optically active substance, because each molecule provides an equal but small contribution to the rotation.

The angle of rotation is normally expressed as specific rotation and mathematically expressed in IP as:

$$\text{Specific rotation} = \frac{\text{Observed rotation (in degrees)}}{\text{Length (dm)} \times \text{density (g/cm}^3)}$$

For liquids : $[\alpha]_D^{25} = \dfrac{\alpha}{1dD^{25}}$

For solids: $[\alpha]_D^{25} = \dfrac{100\,\alpha}{1C}$

where $[\alpha]_D^{25}$ = Specific rotation of a solution at 25 °C

α = corrected rotation at 25 °C, degree

l = length of polarimeter tube, decimetre (dm)

C = concentration of substance, % w/v

d = specific gravity of a liquid or solution at 25 °C

Due to electron vibration plane of plane polarised light changes.

Application

1. Specific rotation is used to identify a substance whether optically active or not. Based on the direction of rotation and magnitude, a substance can be identified (IP).

2. The purity of substance can be measured. It is an important pharmacopoeial test.

3. The concentration of a substance dissolved in a solvent can be determined. This test is used as a quality control test.

4. Polarizability of non polar molecule may be obtained from the measurement of refractive index.

$$\frac{\left(n\,\alpha^2 - 1\right)}{\left(n\,\alpha^2 + 2\right)} \times \frac{M}{\rho} = \frac{4}{3}\pi N \alpha_p$$

From above relationship, induced polarizability p_i can be calculated. In above estimations, relatively 5% error may be incorporated.

5. Refractive index is helpful in calculating the molar refraction without experiment. R_m is used to predict structural features of the molecule.

Determination of Refractive Index

- Several refractometers are available, Abbe's refractometer is a quick and convenient instrument.

Construction

Normally constructed by using white light, but are calibrated to give refractive index in terms of D line of sodium. The apparatus is provided with a water jacket to control the temperature of measurement. Light source should follow as per manufacturer's instructions.

Method

A drop of liquid is placed upon the surface of the prism A. On clamping the prism A and B, the liquid drop spreads as a thin film. Now a mirror M reflects the light and directs towards the prism system. On reaching the ground surface of A, the light is scattered in to the liquid film. A particular ray going along the grazing incidence (at an angle slightly less than 90°) will pass through the prism B at an angle equal to the critical angle (e). According to critical angle phenomenon

$$\sin e = \frac{n}{N}$$

where   n = refractive index of liquid

         N = refractive index of prism

The critical ray emerging from the upper prism at an angle α is viewed by means of telescope. The telescope is fixed and prism box is rotated so as to get coincidence of critical angle with the cross wires of eye pieces. Prism should be setted to a definite critical angle.

When viewed through telescope, the field of view is divided into bright and dark portions. When the edges of bright portion coincide with the cross-wire of the telescope, the scale reading gives the refractive index of the liquids.

The relation between dielectric constant and refractive index is given by-

$$\epsilon = \eta_\alpha^2$$

n_α refractive index of the liquid at higher wave length

ϵ dielectric constant

1. By using refractive index value we can determine dielectric constant
2. Useful in determining molar polarizability.

     where $\epsilon = n_\alpha^2$

$$p_i = \left(\frac{\epsilon - 1}{\epsilon + 2}\right)\frac{M}{\rho} = \frac{4}{3}\pi N \propto p$$

$$p_i = \left(\frac{n_\alpha^2 - 1}{n_\alpha^2 + 2}\right)\frac{M}{\rho} = \frac{4}{3}\pi N \propto p$$

     where p_i = molar polarization

3. By using refractive index we can determine induced polarizability.

Applications

1. Refractive index is used to identify a substance
2. Purity of a substance can be measured (pharmacopoeial standards).
3. Concentration of a substance dissolved in a liquid can be determined (quality control test, assays).
4. The dielectric constant is greatest when dipolar inter action with light is large.

By increase in temperature decrease in refractive index takes place. Velocity decreases.

$$n \, \alpha \, \frac{1}{T}$$

$$n \, \alpha \, \frac{1}{\lambda}$$

Refractive index is inversely proportional to the above.

The molar refractions, R_m is related to both the refractive index and the molecular properties of a compound being tested. It is expressed as per Lorentz and Lorentz as

$$R_m = \frac{n^2 - 1}{n^2 + 2}\left(\frac{M}{\rho}\right)$$

R_m = molar refraction

M = Molecular weight, g/mol

ρ = density of the compound g/ml

n = refractive index

R_m value of compound can often be predicted from the structural features of the molecule.

Each constituent atom or group contributes a portion to the final R_m value as discussed.

- Molar refraction is independent of temperature.
- We can determine molar refraction directly.

It gives information about refractive index and structure of molar compound.

E.g., Ethyl	Methyl	Ketone		n values
		CH_3—CH_2—$\overset{\overset{O}{\|\|}}{C}$—$CH_3$	H $\rightarrow$	1.100
H $\rightarrow$ 8	8 × 1.1		C-C $\rightarrow$	2.418
C-C $\rightarrow$ 3	3 × 2.4		C=C $\rightarrow$	1.733
C = O $\rightarrow$ 1	1 × 2.211	= 18.211	C=C $\rightarrow$	2.211
			(OH) $\rightarrow$	1.525

3.7 Optical Rotation of Chemical Compound

The chemical nature of a substance is mainly responsible for exhibiting the optical activity. These are as follows:

1. Molecules that have an asymmetric centre (chiral) about a single plane are optically active. Chiral centre or chiral carbon is a carbon atom attached by four different groups.

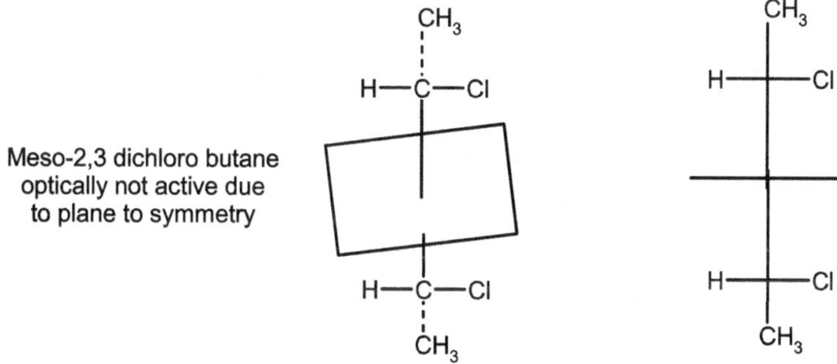

2. Percentage purity of the substance can be determined.

3. Biological activity of drug. E.g., Adrenaline

   - If dextro rotary cannot perform optical action.

   - If Levo rotary can perform optical action.

4. Though the compound possess chiral centres, because of symmetry, the compound losses optical activity.

Factor Influencing Specific Rotation

Specific rotation depends on temperature (t) and wavelength of light source (λ). Normally light source is mercury vapour lamp or sodium lamp, 589 nm.

Optical rotation, α, depends on the density of an optically active substance because each molecule provides an equal but small contribution to the rotation.

The specific rotation. $\left\{\alpha_\lambda^t\right\}$ at a specified temperature t and wave length λ is characteristic for pure, optically active substance. It is given by the equation.

$$\left\{\alpha_\lambda^t\right\} = \frac{\alpha\, v}{lg}$$

l is the length in decimetres (dm)

g is the no. of gm of optically active substance in V millimetre of volume.

Method of Determination of Optical Activity

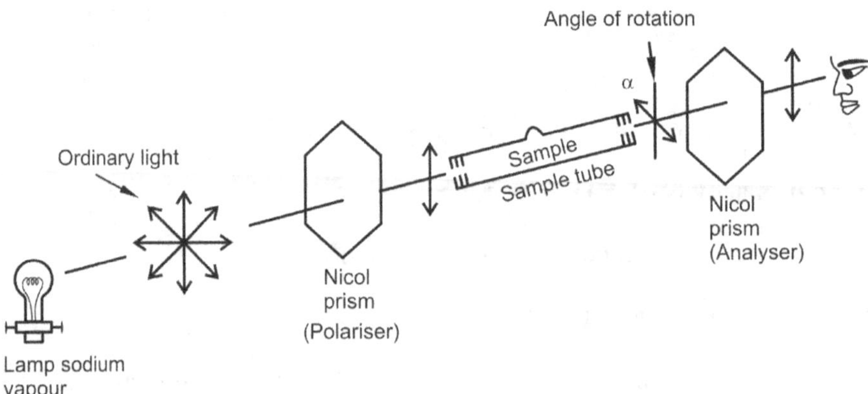

Fig. 3.4

Optical activity is measured using polarimeter. Polarimeter consists of two polarizing elements, one is polariser and the other is an analyser (Fig. 3.4). It is rotated and mounted within a graduated circular scale in order to measure its orientation with respect to the polariser. When the planes of polarization of the two elements are mutually perpendicular, no light is transmitted through the system.

Liquid can be directly filled in the sample tube. If the substance is a solid, accurately weighed portion is transferred into a volumetric flask and dissolved in H_2O or other solvent, as specified. A portion of the solvent is used for blank determination.

The light source is a sodium vapour lamp. Sample between the polarizing elements, the balance is distributed. Analyser must be turned. The scale reading indicates the angle of rotation. The direction of rotation and specific rotation is reported together for a given substance in a given solvent.

3.8 Optical Rotary Dispersion

Optical rotary dispersion is the measure of the angle of rotation as a function of the wave length. Varying the wave length of light, changes the specific rotation for an optically active substance due to electronic structure of the molecule. A graph of specific rotation verses wavelength shows an inflection and then passes through zero at the wavelength of maximum absorption of polarized light. This change in specific rotation is known as cotton effect. Compounds whose specific rotations show a maximum before passing through zero as the wavelength of polarized light becomes smaller are said to show a positive cotton effect, where as if $\{\alpha\}$ shows a maximum after passing through zero, the compound shows a negative cotton effect. Enantiomers can be characterized by the cotton effect; in addition, ORD is often useful for the structural examination of organic compounds.

Problems

Polarizability of Chloroform

1. Chloroform has a molecular weight of 119 g/mole and a density of 1.43 g/cm^3 at 25 °C. What is its induced molar polarizability?

    We have

Sol.
$$p_i = \frac{(\varepsilon - 1)}{(\varepsilon + 2)} \times \frac{M}{\rho}$$
$$= \frac{(4.8 - 1)}{(4.8 + 2)} \times \frac{119}{1.43} = 46.5 \, \text{cm}^3 / \text{mole}$$

3. A solution of lysine containing 1 g/50 ml of 6N HCl was placed in a 40 cm tube in a polarimeter. It had an optical rotation of 1.652°. Calculate the specific rotation of lysine.

Sol.   Data :
$$\alpha = 1.652°$$
$$C = 1 \, \text{g/50 ml} = 2 \, \text{g/100 ml}$$
$$l = 40 \, \text{cm} = 4 \, \text{dm}$$
$$[\alpha] = \frac{100 \, \alpha}{lC} = \frac{100 \times 1.652}{4 \times 2} = 20.65$$

4. The specific rotation of alanine is +14.7°. If its optical rotation in a 20 cm tube is + 1.7°, what is the concentration of alanine in the solution.

Sol.   Date
$$[\alpha] = 14.7°$$
$$\alpha = 1.7°$$
$$l = 20 \, \text{cm} = 2\text{dm};$$
$$C = ?$$

$$[\alpha] = \frac{100\,\alpha}{lC} \qquad \text{(or)} \qquad C = \frac{100\,\alpha}{1 \times [\alpha]}$$

$$C = \frac{100 \times 1.7}{2 \times 14.7} = 5.78 \text{ g/100 ml.}$$

Optical rotary Dispersion

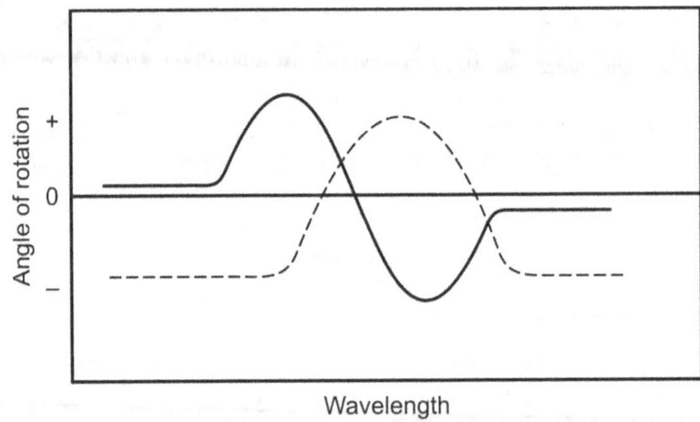

Fig. 3.5 The cotton effect.

Variation of the angle of rotation in the vicinity of an absorption band of polorized light.

Optical Rotatory Dispersion Curves

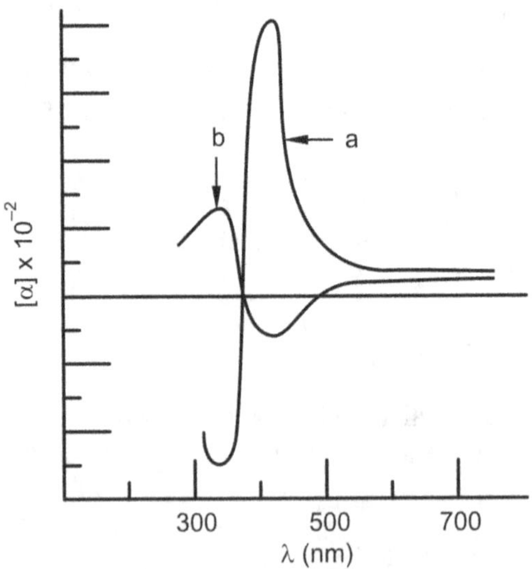

Fig. 3.6 Optical rotary dispersion curves for
(a) Cis-10-methyl-2-decalone (b) Trans-10-methy-2-decalone

Table 3.1 Dipole moment of some compounds.

Compound	Dipole moment (debye units)
P-dichlorobenzene	O
H_2	O
CO_2	O
Benzene	O
1,4-dioxane	O
Carbon monoxide	0.12
Hydrogen iodide	0.38
Hydrogen bromide	0.78
Hydrogen chloride	1.03
Di methyl amine	1.03
Barbital	1.10
Pheno barbital	1.16
Ethylamine	1.22
Formic acid	1.4
Acetic acid	1.4
Phenol	1.45
Ammonia	1.46
m-dichlorobenzene	1.5
Tetra hydrofuron	1.63
n-propanol	1.68
Chloro benzene	1.69
Ethanol	1.69
Methanol	1.70
Dehydro cholesterol	1.81
Water	1.84
Chloroform	1.86
Cholesterol	1.99
Ethylene diamine	1.99
Acetyl salicylic acid	2.07
O-dechloro benzene	2.3
Acetone	2.88
Hydrogen cyanide	2.93

Table 3.1 *Contd...*

Compound	Dipole moment (debye units)
Nitro methane	3.46
Acetanilide	3.55
Androsterone	3.70
Acetonitrile	3.92
Methyl testosterone	4.17
Testosterone	4.32
Urea	4.56
Sulfanilamide	5.37

Table 3.2 Polarizabilities

Molecule	$\alpha_p \times 10^{24}$ (cm^3)
H_2O	1.68
N_2	1.79
HCl	3.01
H Br	3.5
HI	5.6
HCN	5.9

Table 3.3 Dielectric constants of some liquids at 25 ^{o}C

Substance	Dielectric constant, ε
N-methyl formamide	182
Hydrogen cyanide	114
Formamide	110
Water	78.5
Glycerol	42.5
Methanol	32.6
Tetra methyl urea	23.1
Acetone	20.7
n-propanol	20.1
Iso propanol	18.3
Iso pentanol	14.7
I-pentanol	13.9
Benzyl alcohol	13.1
Phenol	9.8 (60 ^{o}C)
Ethyl acetate	6.02

Chloroform	4.80
HCl	4.60
Di ethyl ether	4.34
Acetonitrile	3.92
Carbon disulfide	2.64
Tri ethyl amine	2.42
Toulene	2.38
Bees wax (solid)	2.8
Benzene	2.27
Carbon tetrachloride	2.23
1, 4 Dioxane	2.21
Pentane	1.84 (20 $^{\circ}$C)
Furfural	41 (20 $^{\circ}$C)
Pyridine	12.3
Mathyl salicylate	9.41 (30 $^{\circ}$C)

Table 3.4 Atomic and group contributions to molar refraction.

C-(single)	2.418
-C = (double)	1.733
-C $\equiv$ (triple)	2.398
Phenol ($C_6 H_5$)	25.463
H	1.100
O(C = O)	2.211
O(O-H)	1.525
O (ether, ester, C-O)	1.643
Cl	5.967
Br	8.865
I	13.900

3.9 Questions

1. Describe the principle, construction and working of Abbe's refractometer.

2. Write a detail note on di-electric constant.

3. Enumerate the term Refractive Index and Molar Refraction. Write its importance in pharmacy.

CHAPTER 4

SOLUTIONS OF NON-ELECTROLYTES

4.1 Introduction

Materials can be mixed together to form solution. These solutions may be of three different kinds:

(a) True solution

(b) Coarse dispersion

(c) Colloidal solution

(a) ***True solution:*** It is defined as a mixture of two or more components that form a homogenous molecular dispersion i.e., one phase system.

The term *phase* is defined as a distinct homogenous part of a system separated by different boundaries from other parts of a system.

E.g., 1: Sugar dissolved in water.

E.g., 2: A single piece of ice floating on water.

82

(b) *Coarse dispersion:* In this type of solution the diameter of the particles in solutions range between or larger than 0.1 mm (100 A° (or) 10^{-5} cm)

E.g., Water/other vehicle distributed as oil droplets in suspension or emulsion.

(c) *Colloidal solution:* In these types of solutions the diameter of particles is intermediate between true solution and coarse dispersion (10 – 5000 A°).

A colloidal dispersion may be homogenous (one phase or Heterogeneous (two phase system).

Heterogeneous colloidal solution

E.g., A colloidal dispersion of Acacia/sodium CMC in water. Because it consists if distinct particles as a separate phase.

Homogeneous colloidal solution

E.g., A colloidal dispersion of Acacia/sodium CMC in water

A solution composed of only two substances is known as Binary solutions and its components as solute and solvent.

Solute is the constituent present in lesser amounts in a binary solution, whereas the solvent conversely is the constituent present in large amounts.

Different properties of a binary solution:
 (a) Additive properties
 (b) Constitutive properties
 (c) Intermediate properties
 (d) Colligative properties

(a) *Additive properties:* Depend on total contribution of atoms in the molecule or on the sum of the properties of the constituents in solution.

E.g., Molecular weight i.e., the sum of masses of individual components.

(b) *Constitutive properties:* Depend on the kind of arrangement, number and kind of atoms within a molecule. These properties give information about the constitution of an individual compound and group of molecules in the system.

(c) **Intermediate properties:** These properties (physical properties) are partly additive and constitutive.

E.g., Refraction of light, electric properties, surface and interfacial characteristics etc.

(d) *Colligative properties:* Depend on the number of particles in a solution.

E.g., Osmotic pressure,

Lowering of vapour pressure

Depression of freezing point

Elevation of boiling point

The values of the colligative properties are approximately similar for equal concentrations of different non-electrolytes in solution regardless of the species/chemical nature of the constituents.

Types of Solution: Solution can be classified according to the states in which the solute and solvent occur and because 3 states of matter, occur and 9 types of homogeneous mixtures of solute and solvent are possible.

Types of Solutions

Solute	Solvent	Example
Gas	Gas	Air
Liquid	Gas	Water in oxygen
Solid	Gas	Iodine vapour in air
Gas	Liquid	Carbonated water
Liquid	Liquid	Alcohol in water
Solid	Liquid	Aq. Nacl solution
Gas	Solid	H_2 in palladium
Liquid	Solid	Mineral oil in paraffin
Solid	Solid	Ag-Au mixture Mixture of alums i.e., Alloys

The solutes are divided into (a) Non-electrolytes

(b) Electrolytes

Non-electrolytes: Are the substances that don't yield ions when dissolved in water and therefore don't conduct electric current through the solution.

E.g., Sucrose

Glycerine

Napthalene

Urea......,

For these kinds of solutes the colligative properties are fairly regular.

Electrolytes: Are the substances that form ions in solution, conduct electric current but show anomalous colligative properties.

E.g., Hydrochloric acid

Sodium sulphate

Ephedrine

Phenobarbitol

These electrolytes can be further divided based on their degree of ionization in water.

(a) Strong electrolytes.

(b) Weak electrolytes

4.2 Method of Expressing the Concentration of Solutions

The concentration of a solution can be expressed in terms of quantity of solute in a definite volume of the solution or as a quantity of solute in a definite mass of solvent/solution.

Molarity: It is defined as the no. of moles i.e., gram molecular weights of solute present in 1 litre solution.

It is represented as M (or) C

$$M = \text{no. of moles of solute} \times 1/V \text{ unit solution}$$

$$= \frac{\text{weight}}{\text{Gram molecular weight}} \times \frac{1000}{V \text{ in ml}}$$

Normality: It is defined as the number of gram equivalent weights of solute in 1 lt solution.

It is represented as N

$$N = \frac{\text{weight}}{\text{Gram. equivalent weight}} \times \frac{1000}{V \text{ in ml}}$$

Both the molar and normal solutions are popular in chemistry because representing a known weight of the solute and bringing to the convenient volume is easily obtained by use of burette or pipette.

Note: But, both molarity and normality have the disadvantage of changing value with temperature because of the expansion/contraction of liquids and therefore it should not be used when one desires to study properties of solutions at different temperatures.

Molality: It is defined as the number of moles of solute present in 1000 g of solvent.

As it is based on the terms of 'weight' it don't have any errors as discussed earlier in case of different temperatures. It is representing as 'm'.

$$m = \frac{\text{weight of solute}}{\text{Gram. molecular weight of solute}} \times \frac{1000}{'a' \text{ in gm}}$$

where a = weight of solvent in 'g'

Molefraction: It is defined as the ratio of the moles of one constituent (E.g., solute of a solution) to the total moles of all constituents (both the solute and solvent). It is represented by X (or) N

It is expressed as:

$$X_1 = \frac{n_1}{n_1 + n_2}$$

$$X_2 = \frac{n_2}{n_1 + n_2}$$

where

X_1 = mole refraction of solute

X_2 = mole refraction of solvent

n_1 = no. of moles of solute

n_2 = no. of moles of solvent

Percentage Expressions

It may again be of 3 types

Percent by weight

Percent by volume

Percent weight in volume

Percent by weight (% w/w): It is number of grams of solute in 100 g of solution.

Percent by volume (% v/v): It is number of millilitres of solute in 100 ml of solution.

Percent weight in volume (% w/v): It is the number of grams of solute in 100 ml of solution.

Problems

1. An aqueous solution of exsiccated $FeSO_4$ was prepared adding 41.50 g of $FeSO_4$ to enough water to make 1000 ml of solution of 18 °C. The density of solution is 1.0375 and its molecular weight is 151.9 g. Calculate (a) the molarity; (b) molality; (c) the mole fraction of $FeSO_4$, the mole fraction of water and the mole percent of two constituents; and (d) the percentage by weight of $FeSO_4$.

Sol.　(a) Molarity

$$\text{Moles of } FeSO_4 = \frac{\text{g of } FeSO_4}{\text{Gmw of } FeSO_4} = \frac{41.50}{151.9} = 0.2732 \text{ moles}$$

$$\text{Molarity} = \frac{\text{Moles of } FeSO_4}{\text{Litres of solution}} = \frac{0.2732}{1} = 0.2732 \text{ M}$$

(b) Molality

Grams of solution $= \text{Volume} \times \text{Density}$

$$= 1000 \times 1.0375$$

$$= 1037.5 \text{ g}$$

Gram of solvent $= \text{Grams of solution} - \text{gms of FeSO4}$

$$= 1037.5 - 41.5$$

$$= 996.0 \text{ g}$$

$$\text{Molality} = \frac{\text{Moles of FeSO}_4}{1000 \text{ g of solvent}} = \frac{0.2732}{0.996} = 0.2743 \text{ m}$$

(c) Mole fraction and mole percent

$$\text{Moles of water} = \frac{996.0}{18.02} = 55.27 \text{ moles}$$

Mole fraction of $FeSO_4 =$

$$X_2 = \frac{\text{Moles of FeSO}_4}{\text{Moles of water} + \text{moles of FeSO}_4} = \frac{0.2732}{55.27 + 0.2732}$$

$$= 0.0049$$

Mole fraction of water $=$

$$X_1 = \frac{\text{Moles of water}}{\text{Moles of water} + \text{Moles of FeSO}_4} = \frac{55.27}{55.27 + 0.2732}$$

$$= 0.9951$$

Notice that.

$$X_1 + X_2 = 0.9951 + 0.0049 = 1.0000$$

Mole percent of $FeSO_4 = 0.0049 \times 100 = 0.49\%$

Mole percent of water $= 0.9951 \times 100 = 99.51\%$

(d) Percentage by weight of $FeSO_4$:

$$= \frac{\text{g of FeSO}_4}{\text{g of solution}} \times 100$$

$$= \frac{41.50}{1037.5} \times 100$$

$$= 4.00\%$$

Conversion Equations for Concentration Terms

(a) Molality (moles of solute/kg of solvent, m) and mole fraction of solute (X_2)

$$X_2 = \frac{m}{m + \dfrac{1000}{M_1}}$$

$$m = \frac{1000\,X_2}{M_1\left(1-X_2\right)} = \frac{1000\left(1-X_1\right)}{M_1 X_1}$$

(b) Molarity (moles of solute/litre of solution, C) and mole fraction of solute (X_2)

$$X_2 = \frac{C}{C + \dfrac{1000\rho - C\,M_2}{M_1}}$$

$$C = \frac{1000\,\rho X_2}{M_1\left(1-X_2\right) + M_2\,X_2}$$

(c) Molality (m) and molarity (C):

$$m = \frac{1000\,C}{1000\,\rho - M_2 C}$$

$$C = \frac{1000\,\rho}{\dfrac{1000}{m} + M_2}$$

(d) Molality (m) and molarity (C) in terms of weight of solute w_2, weight of solvent w_1, molecular weight M_2 of solute.

$$m = \frac{w_2/M_2}{w_1/1000} = \frac{1000\,w_2}{w_1\,M_2}$$

$$C = \frac{1000\,\rho w_2}{M_2\left(w_1 + w_2\right)}$$

4.3 Ideal and Real Solutions

Ideality in a gas implies the complete absence of attraction forces, ideality in a solution means complete uniformity of attractive forces. Because a liquid is a highly condensed state, it cannot be expected to be devoid of attractive forces; nevertheless, if, is a mixture of A & B molecules, the forces between A and A, B and B and A and B are all of the same order and the solution is said to be ideal.

Ideal solution: is defined as the one in which there is no change in properties of the components other than dilution, when they are mixed to form a solution.

- No heat should be evolved or absorbed during the process of mixing.
- The final volume of the solution represents an additive property of individual constituents i.e., no shrinkage or expansion occurs when the substances are mixed.

Ideal solutions are formed by mixing substances with similar properties. For e.g., when 100 ml of methanol is mixed with 100 ml of ethanol, the final volume of the solution is 200 ml and no heat is evolved or absorbed. The solution is nearly ideal.

Real solution/non-ideal solution: are defined as the solutions which don't behave as ideal solutions. For e.g., when 100 ml of sulphuric acid is combined with 100 ml of water, however, the volume of the solution is about 180 ml at room temperature, and the mixing is by a considerable evolution of heat.

Raoult's law

The vapour pressure of liquid serves as a quantitative expression for describing the escaping tendencies of molecules.

Statement: Raoult's law states that the partial vapour pressure of each volatile constituent is equal to the vapour pressure of the pure constituent multiplied by its molefraction in the solution, at a given temperature.

Since the solution is homogenous, the relative number components on the surface reflect the numbers of components in whole of the solution. These numbers can be expressed on the molefraction scale.

This law is suited to describe the ideal solution.

Consider a mixture of miscible liquids A & B. In this mixture:

Let partial vapour pressure exerted by liquid A $= P_A$ KP_a

Let partial vapour pressure exerted by liquid B $= P_B$ KP_a

Let vapour pressure exerted by pure liquid A $= P_A^o$ KP_a

Let vapour pressure exerted by pure liquid B $= P_B^o$ KP_a

Let mole fraction concentration of A in liquid $= X_A$

Let mole fraction concentration of B in liquid $= X_B$

Raoutls law may be mathematically expressed as:

Partial vapour pressure of a liquid = Vapour pressure of pure liquid × Mole fraction of Liquid

$$P_A = P_A^o \, X_A$$

$$P_B = P_B^o \, X_B$$

For e.g., if the vapour pressure of the ethylene chloride in the pure state is 236 mm Hg at 50 °C, then in a solution consisting of a mole fraction of 0.4 ethylene chloride and 0.6 benzene, the partial V.P of ethylene chloride is 40% of 236 mm, or 94.4 mm. Thus, in an ideal solution, when liquid A is mixed with B, the V.P of A is mixed with B in a manner depending on the mole fractions of A & B present in the final solution. This will diminish escaping tendency of each constituent, leading to a reduction in the rate of escape of molecules of A & B from surface of liquid.

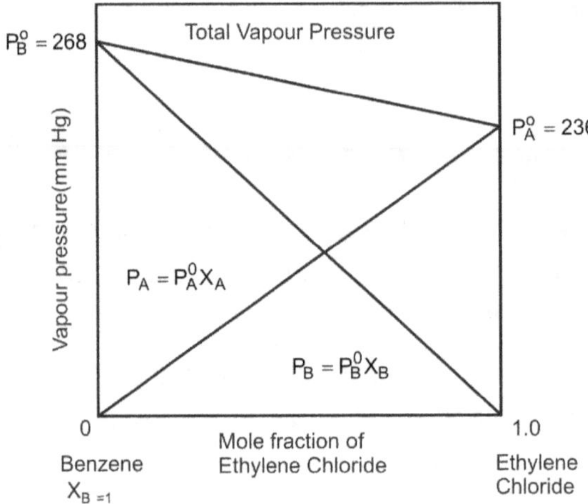

Fig. 4.1 Vapour pressure – composition curve for an ideal binary system.

Real solutions which don't follow the Raoult's law exhibit two types of deviations:

(a) Positive deviation

(b) Negative deviation

Positive deviation: In some liquids, the vapour pressure is greater than the sum of partial pressures of the individual components, such systems are said to exhibit positive deviation from Raoult's law.

E.g., Carbon tetrachloride and cyclohexane

Benzene and ethanol

Water and ethanol

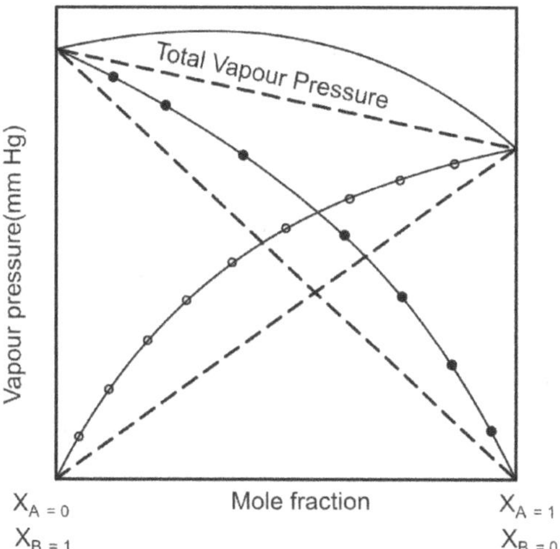

Fig. 4.2 Vapour pressure of a system showing positive deviation from Roult's law.

In this, the interaction between A & B molecules is less than that between molecules of pure constituents, the presence of 'B' molecules reduces the interaction of the 'A' molecules, and 'A' molecules correspondingly reduces the B-B interaction.

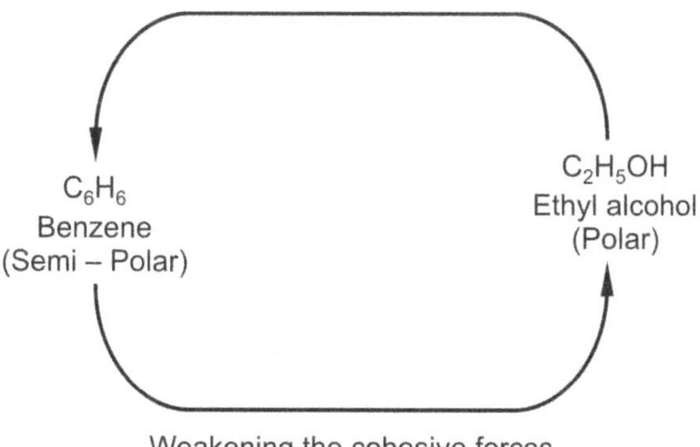

Weakening the cohesive forces

Negative deviation: In some liquid systems, the vapour pressure is less than the sum of partial pressures of the individual components. Such systems are said to exhibit negative deviation from Raoult's law.

When the 'adhesive' attractions between molecules between molecules of different species exceed the "cohesive" attraction between like molecules, the V.P of solution is less than expected from Raoult's ideal solution law and negative deviation occurs.

E.g., Chloroform and acetone
  (A)   (B)

The dilution of constituent A by addition of B normally would be expected to reduce the partial pressure of A.

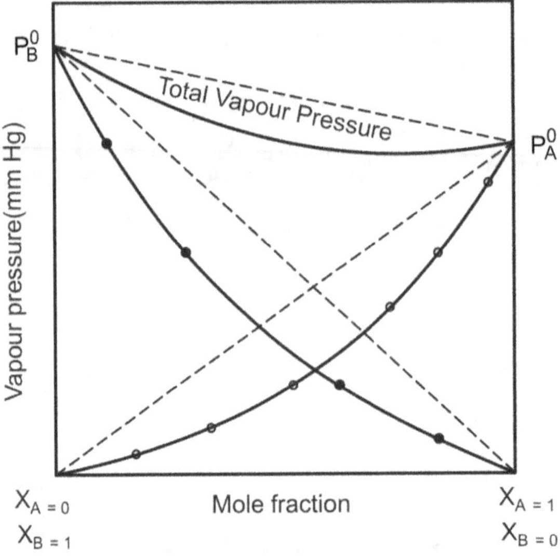

In the chloroform and Acetone due to H-bonding, the adhesive forces dominate than cohesive forces, thus further reducing the escaping tendency of each constituent. This pair forms a weak compound.

Fig 4.3 Vapour pressure of a system showing negative deviation from Raoult's law.

4.4 Colligative Properties

The freezing point, boiling point and osmotic pressure of a solution also depend on the relative proportion of the molecules of the solute and solvent. These are called colligative properties (Greek: Collected together) because they depend chiefly on the number of molecules rather than its constituents.

Applications

Colligative properties have a number of applications. Among them, osmotic pressure has the greatest important in pharmacy, because it determines the physiological acceptability of a solution.

1. Molecular mass of a substance can be determined

2. We can determine whether the solution is iso-osmotic or not

3. Dosage forms of such as injections, eye drops and nasal drops i.e., isotonic solutions are prepared. The Nacl equivalents of drugs are determined based on the colligative properties. The equivalents can be used for the calculation of composition while preparing the isotonic solutions.

4. The behaviour of solution of electrolytes can be understood.

5. The osmotic properties of body fluids such as lacrimal fluids and blood are evaluated. These are useful in understanding the phenomenon of haemolysis.

4.4.1 Lowering of Vapour Pressure

When a non-volatile solute is added to a solvent, solvent molecules solely provide vapour pressure above the solution. The vapour pressure of the solution is decreased, when compared to that of a pure solvent.

Let vapour pressure of the pure solvent $= P_1^o \ KP_a$

Let vapour pressure of the solution $= P \ KP_a$

Lowering of vapour pressure, $\Delta P = \left(P_1^o - P \right) KP_a$

Relative lowering of vapour pressure (RLVP) $= \dfrac{P_1^o - P}{Pi} = \dfrac{\Delta P}{P_1^o}$

Raoult gave the relationship between the RLVP and the concentration of the solute in solution.

Raoult's law of RLVP states that the RLVP of a solute solution is equal to the mole fraction of the solute present in solution.

It is expressed as $\dfrac{\Delta P}{P_1^o} = X_2 = \dfrac{n_2}{n_1 + n_2}$

n_2 = number of moles of solute

n_1 = number of moles of solvent

Relative lowering of vapour pressure is dimensionless number.

Derivation of Raoult's Law

The vapourization of solvent molecules from a pure solvent and a solution. In case of pure-solvent, vapour pressure is due to the escaping of a number of solvent molecules from its surfaces. When a non-volatile solute is dissolved in the solution, the solute molecules in the surface block a fraction of the surface so that solvent evaporation decreases. This causes the lowering of the vapour-pressure.

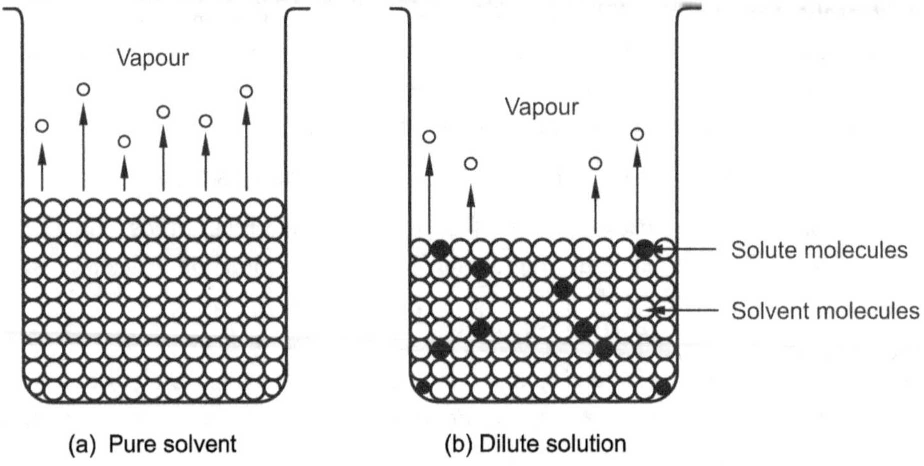

Fig. 4.4 The effect of non-volatile solute on vapour pressure of the solvent.

Limitations of Raoult's law of lowering of vapour pressure: An ideal solution is one, which follows Raoutlt's law over the entire range of concentrations. While applying Raout's law to real solution, it has following limitations.

Dilute solutions: Raoult's law is applicable to dilute solutions because intermolecular attractions are nil or weak. When the concentration of the solute is high, intermolecular forces gain prominence and cause deviation.

Non-volatile solutes: The law is applicable to solutions containing non-volatile solute. If the solute is volatile, it also contributes to vapour pressure. This cause deviation in lowering of vapour-pressure.

No dissociation of molecules: Raoults law does not apply if the solute dissociates.

E.g., $\quad AB \rightarrow A^+ + B^-$

In this the solute dissociates into ions which act as individual molecule and because of this the V.P will become twice that of the original.

No association of molecules: Raoult's law does not apply for the molecules which get associated into one compound because of which the vapour pressure becomes half of the expected.

E.g., $\qquad 2A \rightarrow A_2$

Determination of Molecular Mass for Lowering of Vapour Pressure

From the lowering of vapour pressure ($P_1^o - P$), the molecular mass of a non-volatile solute can be determined. When a solute is dissolved in solvent,

$$\text{Number of moles of solute} = \frac{\text{Weight of solute}}{\text{Molecular mass of the solute}}$$

$$n_2 = \frac{w_2}{M_2} \qquad \qquad \text{.....(4.1)}$$

$$\text{Number of moles of solvent} = \frac{\text{Weight of solvent}}{\text{Molecular mass of solvent}}$$

$$n_2 = \frac{w_1}{M_1} \qquad \qquad \text{.....(4.2)}$$

Substituting eq. (4.1) and (4.2) in the Raoult's law equation gives

$$\frac{\Delta P}{P_1^o} = \frac{n_2}{n_1 + n_2} = \frac{\left(w_2/M_2\right)}{\left(\dfrac{w_1}{M_1}\right) + \left(\dfrac{w_2}{M_2}\right)} \qquad \qquad \text{.....(4.3)}$$

In dilute solution, the number of moles of solute (w_2/M_2) is very small; it can be neglected in denominator. The above equation (4.3) can be written as:

$$\frac{\Delta P}{P_1^o} = \frac{\left(w_2/M_2\right)}{\left(w_1/M_1\right)}$$

$$\frac{\Delta P}{P_1^o} = \frac{w_2\, M_1}{w_1\, M_2}$$

On rearranging

$$M_2 = \frac{w_2\, M_1\, P_1^o}{\Delta P\, w_1}$$

where

M_2 = molecular mass of solute, g/mol

M_1 = molecular mass of solvent, g/mol

ΔP = lowering of vapour pressure, P_a

P_1^o = vapour pressure of solvent, KP_a

w_2 = weight of solute, g

w_1 = weight of solvent, g

Relationship between relative lowering of vapour pressure and molality: In dilute solutions, mole fractions solubility of solute (X_2) and molality (m) can be written as:

$$\frac{n_2}{n_1 + n_2} = X_2 = 0.018\,m$$

According to Raoult's law of RLVP, the relationship may be expressed as

$$\frac{\Delta P}{P_1^o} = 0.018\,m$$

Measurement of Lowering of Vapour Pressure

The vapour pressure of the solvent and solution may be directly measured by means of a manometer. Differential manometers can be used for the accurate measurement of small differences in pressures. The isopiestic method is described here for the precise determination of vapour pressure.

Isopiestic Method

The apparatus for isopiestic method is shown in Fig. 4.5. The solution whose vapour pressure should be determined is placed in a dish and kept in a closed container. Along with it, a dish containing a solution of standard solute, for E.g., KCl, is placed. The container is evacuated to hasten the vapourization and achieving rapid equilibrium. The vapour of the solution with the higher pressure passes to the one with lower pressure. This process continues until the vapour pressure of both become equal i.e., isopiestic (Greek: equal pressures) when there is no change in weight, the solutions are analysed to determine their concentrations.

The initial and final pressure (same as the vapour pressure of the test solution) of the potassium chloride (KCl) are determined accurately using tables available in the literature. From these, vapour pressure of test solution is obtained knowing the vapour pressure of water at this temperature, lowering of vapour pressure of solution can be calculated.

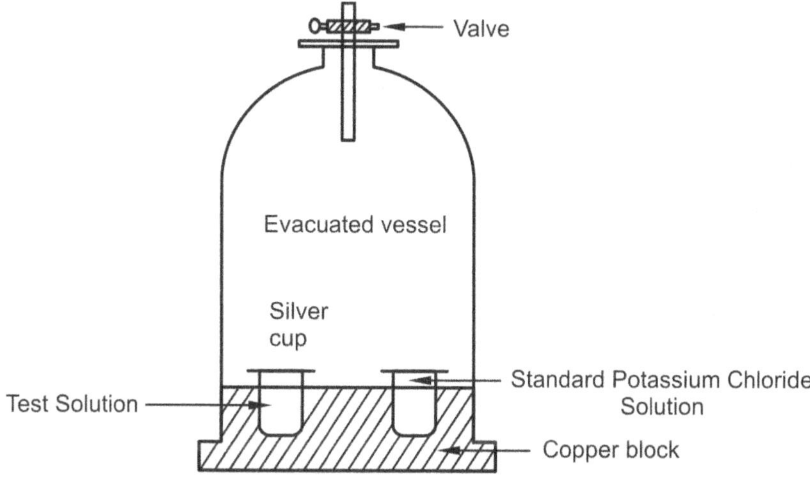

Fig. 4.5 Appratus for the Isopiestic method.

There is also other apparatus called Hills and Blades apparatus consisting essentially of a combination of various wires of different alloys formed into two loops and connected to a galvanometer as shown in Fig. 4.6 given below for determining the relative vapour pressures of small amounts of liquid. This thermo-electric method depends on measuring the change in potential as a solution of known vapour pressure and an unknown evaporate in a chamber maintained at a constant humidity.

This method is used to study the colligative properties of ophthalmic solutions.

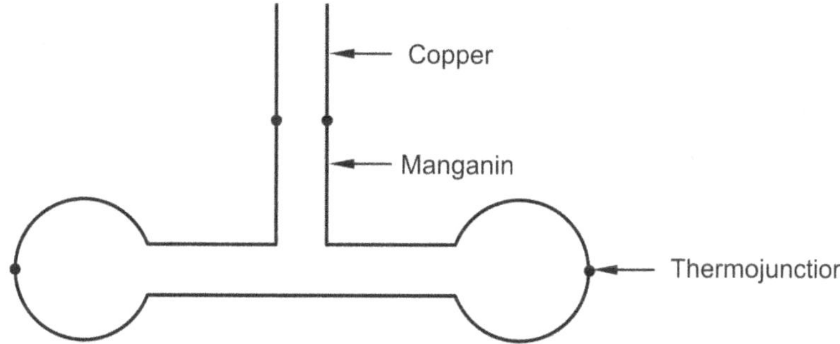

Fig. 4.6 Hill-Baldes apparatus for thermolelectric determination of vapour pressure.

4.4.2 Elevation of Boiling Point

Boiling point of a solvent is the temperature at which the vapour pressure is equal to the atmospheric pressure. The vapour pressure of the solvent is maximum at its boiling point.

When a non-volatile solute is added to the solvent, the vapour pressure is lowered. As a result more heat is to be supplied (higher temperature) in order to make the vapour pressure equal to atmospheric pressure. In other words, the boiling point of the solvent is increased due to the presence of non-volatile solute.

Let, the boiling point of solvent = T_b °C

the boiling point of solution = T °C

Elevation in boiling point, $\Delta T_b = (T - T_b)$ °C

The relationship between the elevation of boiling point and lowering of vapour pressure is shown Fig.

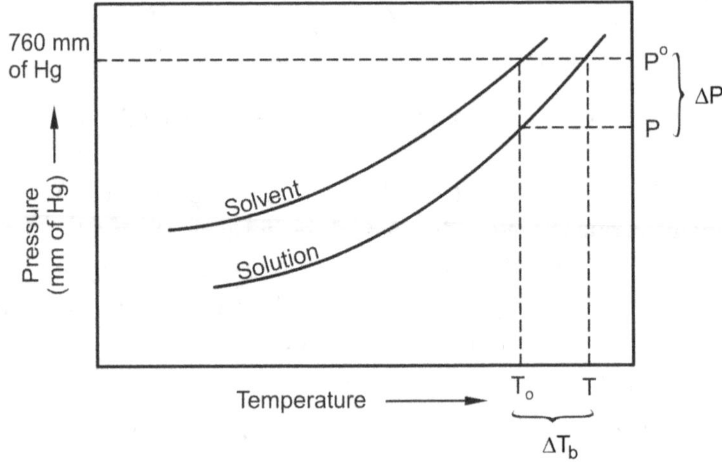

Fig. 4.7 Boiling point elevation of the solvent due to addition of a solute.

The ratio of elevation of boiling point, (ΔT_b), to the vapour pressure lowering, $\Delta P = P^\circ - P$ at 100 °C is approximately a constant at this temperature; it is written as,

$$\frac{\Delta T_b}{\Delta P} = k' \qquad\qquad .....(4.4)$$

or $$\Delta T_b = k'\Delta P$$

Since the P° is a constant, the boiling point elevation may be considered proportional to $\Delta P/P^\circ$ i.e., RLVP.

By Raoult's law, the RLVP is equal to the mole fraction of solute and therefore,

$$\Delta T_b = kX_2 \qquad\qquad .....(4.5)$$

Because the elevation of boiling point is dependent only on the mole fraction of solute, it is a colligative property.

In dilute solution, X_2 is equal to

$$X_2 = \frac{m}{\frac{1000}{M_1}}$$

$$X_2 = \frac{m.M_1}{1000}$$

Substituting in eq. 4.5 with value of X_2 we get,

$$\Delta T_b = k.\frac{m.M_1}{1000}$$

$$\Delta T_b = K_b m$$

where,

ΔT_b = Elevation in boiling point

K_b = Ebullioscopic constant/molal elevation constant

The K_b value is a characteristic for each solvent as seen in below Table 4.1.

Table 4.1 Ebullioscopic and cryoscopic constant for various solvents.

Substance	B.P in (°C)	K_b	F.P. in (°C)	K_f
Acetic acid	118	2.93	16.7	3.9
Benzene	80.1	2.53	5.5	5.12
Camphor	208.3	5.95	178.4	37.7
Ethyl alcohol	78.4	1.22	−144.49	3

K_b ebullioscopic constant is defined as the boiling point elevation for an ideal 1 m solution. i.e., K_b is the ratio of the boiling point elevation to the molal concentration in an extremely dilute solution.

By the application of Claussius-Clapeyron equation the above eq. 4.4 is written as:

$$\frac{\Delta T_b}{\Delta P} = T_b.\frac{V_v - V_l}{\Delta H_v} \qquad\qquad .....(4.6)$$

where

V_V = molar volume of gas

V_l = molar volume of liquid

T_b = boiling point of solvent

ΔH_V = molar heat of vaporisation

In the above eq. 4.6, V_l is negligible compared to V_V so, the equation becomes

$$\frac{\Delta T_b}{\Delta P} = T_b \cdot \frac{V_V}{\Delta H_V}$$

And V_V, the volume of one mole of gas, is replaced by

$$\frac{R\,T_b}{P^o} \qquad\qquad \because P^o V_V = R\,T_b$$

$$V_V = \frac{R\,T_b}{P^o}$$

$$\therefore \qquad \frac{\Delta T_p}{\Delta P} = \frac{R\,T_b^2}{P^o \Delta H_V}$$

or

$$\Delta T_b = \frac{R\,T_b^2}{\Delta H_v} \cdot \frac{\Delta P}{P^o} \qquad\qquad\qquad .....(4.7)$$

By substituting $\dfrac{\Delta P}{P^o} = X_2$ in eq. 4.7 we get,

$$\Delta T_b = \frac{R\,T_b^2}{\Delta H_V}\, X_2 = KX_2 \qquad\qquad\qquad .....(4.8)$$

which provides a more exact equation to calculate ΔT_b.

Also by replacing the X_2 by $\dfrac{M_1 . m}{1000}$, we get

$$\Delta T_b = \frac{R\,T_b^2\,M_1}{1000 . \Delta H_v} . m = K_b . m \qquad\qquad\qquad .....(4.9)$$

Determination of Boiling Point

Boiling point deviation is determined by 2 sets of experiments.

Set 1 : Determination of B.P of solvent

Set 2 : Determination of B.P of solution, after placing a weighted amount of solute in solvent.

Landsberger-Walker Method or Ebullioscopic Method

The apparatus used in this method is shown in Fig. The apparatus consists of following:

(i)   An inner tube with a hole in its side and graduated in (ml) is used to place in solvent or solution.

(ii)   A boiling flask is used for sending solvent vapour into the graduated tube through a rose head (a bulb with several holes).

(iii)   An outer tube is used for receiving hot solvent vapour through the side hole of the inner tube.

(iv)   A thermometer with reading to 0.01 °C is dipped in solvent or solution in the inner tube.

Procedure: Pure solvent (about 10 ml of water) is placed in the graduated tube. The vapour of the same solvent boiling in a separate flask is passes into the graduated tube. The vapour causes the solvent to boil by its latent heat of condensation. When the solvent starts boiling, the temperature remains constant. The boiling point is recorded (T_b).

Now the supply of vapour is temporarily cut off. The solvent in the inner tube is removed. A known amount of solute (about 0.5 g) is quantitatively transferred into a 10 ml solvent. This solution is placed in the inner tube. The solvent vapour is again passed, until the boiling point of solution is reached. The B.P of solution is noted (T). The difference in the boiling points gives elevation of boiling point ($T_b - T = \Delta T_b$), the solvent vapour is then cut off, thermometer and rose head are removed. The volume of solution is recorded. From the density determination, the weight (W) is estimated. The weight of solute is subtracted from the weight of solution to obtain the weight of solvent ($w_1 - w - w_2$).

The values obtained are substituted in the $M_2 = \dfrac{1000\,K_b\,w_2}{w_1\,\Delta T_b}$ to get molecular mass of solute.

Precautions

1.   The liquid should not be superheated.

2.   The boiling point changes with variation of atmospheric pressure.

3.   Temperature shows variation with position of thermometer.

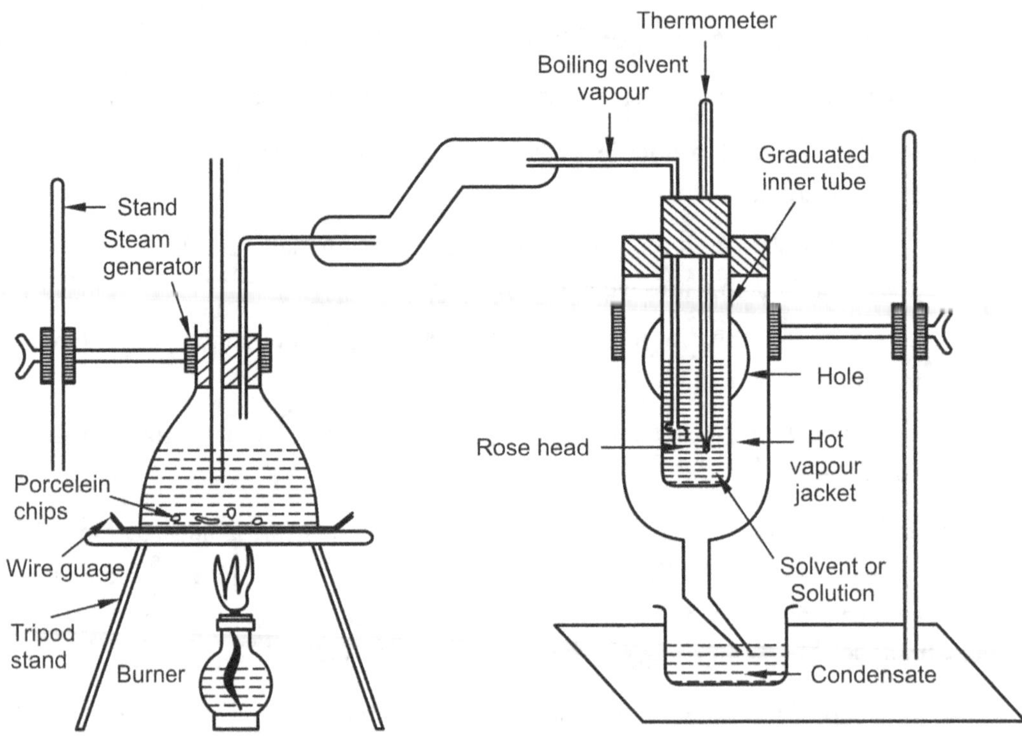

Fig. 4.8 Relationship between vapour pressure and temperature of solvent and solutions.

4.4.3 Depression of Freezing Point

Freezing point or melting point of a pure component is the temperature at which the solid and liquid are in equilibrium at 1 atmosphere (101.3 Kp$_a$).

The freezing point of water is 0 °C. At this temperature the solid and liquid possess same vapour pressure. Here equilibrium means the escaping tendency for the solid to pass into the liquid state is the same as that of the liquid passing into the solid state.

If a solute is dissolved in liquid, the escaping tendency of liquid solvent from solid solution is lowered compared to that of the pure solid solvent. Hence, in order to re-establish equilibrium between the liquid and solid, there is a need to decrease the escaping tendency of molecules from the solid state. This can be achieved by lowering the temperature. Therefore, freezing point of solution is always lower than that of the pure solvent. This is known as freezing point depression.

Let freezing point of the solvent = T_f °C

Let freezing point of the solution = T_A °C

Depression of freezing point due to solution A,

$$\Delta T_f = (T_f - T_A)\ ^{\circ}C$$

The relationships between temperature and vapour pressure of solvent and solutions are shown in Fig. 4.9. CEB curve represents the pure solvent. A sharp break at point B represents the commencement of freezing. This relationship of solution A is shown by curve CFD in following diagram. It is similar to the vapour pressure curve of pure solvent and meets the freezing point curve at F.

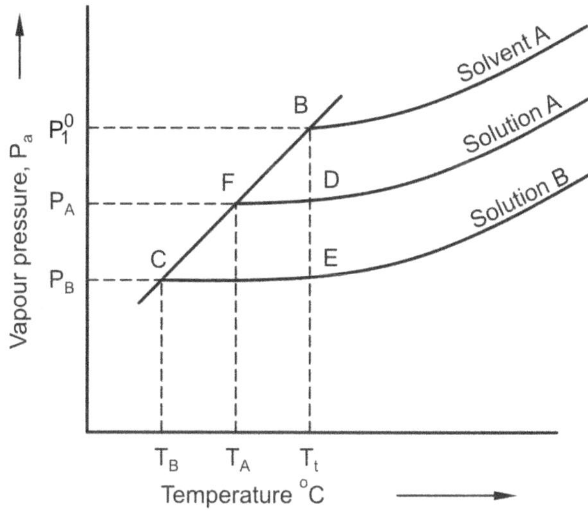

Fig. 4.9 Relationship between vapour pressure and temperature
of solvent and solutions.

When more of the solute is added to the solution A, a more concentrated solution (B) is obtained. The vapour pressure curve of solution B meets the freezing point curve at 'C'.

Depression of freezing point due to solution B,

$$\Delta T_f = (T_F - T_B)\ ^{\circ}C$$

For dilute solutions, FD and CE are approximately parallel and straight lines. BC is a straight line. Since the triangle BDF and BEC are similar, the following relationship can be written.

$$\frac{DF}{EC} = \frac{BD}{BE}$$

$$\frac{T_f - T_A}{T_f - T_B} = \frac{P_1^o - P_A}{P_1^o - P_B}$$

where

P_1^o = vapour pressure of the solvent, K P_a

P_A = Vapour pressure of the solution A KP_a

PB = Vapour pressure of the solution B KP_a

From the above equation it can be represented as:

$$\Delta T_f \alpha \left(P_1^o - P_A \right) \quad \text{(or)} \quad \Delta T_f \alpha \Delta p$$

Determination of Molecular Mass from Depression of Freezing Point

The relationship between the depression of freezing point and lowering of vapour pressure may be written as

$$\Delta T_f \propto \Delta P$$

The higher the concentration of the solute, the greater the freezing point depression. Hence depression of freezing point can be used to determine the molecular mass of solute.

Since P_1^o is constant for a solvent at a fixed temperature, equation can be written as:

$$\Delta T_f \, \alpha \, \frac{\Delta P}{P_1^o}$$

According to Raoult's law $\quad \dfrac{\Delta P}{Pi} = X_2 = \dfrac{m.M_1}{1000}$

$$\Delta T_f = \frac{K.M_1}{1000} .m$$

$$\Delta T_f = K_f.m$$

ΔT_f = molal depression constant (or) cryoscopic constant or freezing point depression constant

The unit of K_f is °C/mol.

Cryoscopic constant is defined as the freezing point depression produced when one mole of solute is dissolved in 1 Kg of the solvent.

According the Classius-Clapeyron, the equation can be written as,

$$\frac{\Delta T_f}{\Delta P} = T_f \frac{V_l - V_S}{\Delta H_f}$$

As in case of elevation of boiling point, we get

$$\Delta T_f = \frac{R\, T_f^2 . M_1}{1000 . \Delta H_f} . m$$

$$\Delta T_f = K_f . m$$

Derivation of molecular weight of solute M_2

$$\Delta T_f = K . m$$

$$\Delta T_f = K_f . \frac{1000 . w_2}{M_2\, w_1} \qquad \because m = \frac{w_2/M_2}{w_1} \times 1000$$

$$M_2 = \frac{K_f}{\Delta T_f} . 1000 . \frac{w_2}{w_1} \qquad = \frac{1000\, w_2}{M_2\, w_1}$$

Measurement of Freezing Point Depression

Similar to the methods of determination of other colligative properties, freezing point depression method also consists of two sets of experiments.

Set 1 : Determination of freezing point of solvent

Set 2 : Determination of freezing point of solution

The most commonly used methods include:

1. Beckmann's method/cryoscopic method
2. Rast camphor method

Beckmann's method/cryoscopic method: The apparatus and assembling for freezing point determination is shown in Fig. It consists of following:

(i) A freezing tube is used to place the solvent/solution. Its side arm helps in introducing the solute into tube.

(ii) An outer large tube is used for fixing the freezing tube. The outer tube acts as an air jacket, which ensures a slow and more uniform rate of cooling.

(iii) A larger jar contains the freezing mixture, for example ice and salt. A stirrer is used for mixing.

Beckmann differential thermometer permits reading up to $\pm\, 0.005\ ^{\circ}C$.

Procedure: About 15-20 g of solvent (say water) is transferred into the freezing tube. The apparatus shown consists of a, bulb of thermometer is completely immersed in the solvent. The mixture is stirred to cool by placing the tube in cooling bath. Then after cooling, it is removed and the external condensate is wiped off. This tube is placed cautiously in air jacket. The temperature is allowed to fall slowly. When the temperature reaches to about 0.5 $^{\circ}C$ below the freezing point, stir vigorously. This causes the solid to separate and the temperature will rise owing to the latent heat set free. The highest temperature is reached and noted down (T_f).

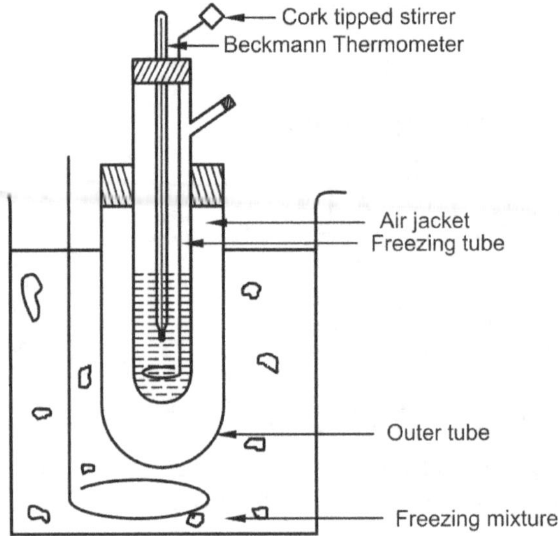

Fig. 4.10 Beckmann's Freezing point apparatus.

The freezing point is removed from the ice bath and allowed to melt. A weighed (about 0.1 – 0.2 g) amount of solute is introduced through the side-tube. Now the M.P if solution (T) is determined in same way as the solvent. A further quantity of solute may be added and another reading is taken.

The depression of the freezing point is calculated ($\Delta T_f = T_f - T$).

The molecular mass of solute is determined using

$$M_2 = \frac{1000 \, K_f \, \omega_2}{\omega_1 \, \Delta T_f}$$

Precautions

(a) Liquid should not be super-cooled, which should not exceed 0.5 $^\circ$C.

(b) Stirring should be uniform at a rate of about one movement per second.

(c) The temperature of the cooling bath should not be 4-5 $^\circ$C below the freezing of the liquid.

(d) If the solvent is crystallised out, the concentration of the solution increases.

(e) While noting the temperature, latent heat liberated on crystallization of solid solvent should be considered

Rast Camphor Method

Camphor can be used as solid solvent, because the freezing point depression is so large (40.0 °C) that the ordinary thermometer is not required. Hence, the Beckmann's thermometer is not used. Another advantage is that ambient conditions can be used. The compound under study should be soluble in molten camphor.

Procedure: Pure camphor is powdered and introduced into a capillary tube, which is sealed at upper end. The M.P of camphor is determined using melting point apparatus. The M.P of camphor is recorded (T_f).

A weighed amount of solute (the substance should be 10 times less than camphor) and camphor are melted in an ampoule with an open end sealed. The mixture is cooled for solidification. The ampoule is broken and the mixture is collected. The solid solution (mixture) is introduced into a capillary tube and sealed at the upper end. The M.P of the mixture is determined (T).

The difference in the melting points gives the depression in the melting point ($\Delta T_f = T_f - T$). The data is substituted in the following equation to calculate molecular mass

$$M_2 = \frac{1000\, K_f\, w_2}{w_1\, \Delta T_f}$$

4.4.4 Osmotic Pressure

Osmosis is defined as a process in which the solvent molecules pass through a semi-permeable membrane from a pure solvent to a solution or from a dilute solution to a concentrated solution.

The process of osmosis proceeds to equalize the concentrations in contact with each other. Thus, equilibrium is achieved.

Semi-permeable membrane is a barrier, which selectively permits the passage of solvent molecules, but not the solute molecules. A few semi-permeable membranes are:

- Animal/pig bladder
- Cellophane
- membranes of RBC's

Application

(a) Osmotic pressure principles are used in the preparation of isotonic intravenous and isotonic lacrimal fluids. Such solutions are compatible to body fluids and prevent the damage of delicate membranes.

(b) In experimental physiology, the tissue is immersed in salt-solutions, which are isotonic. Other wise, tissue gets damaged due to osmosis.

(c) Extent of ionisation can be determined in case of electrolytes.

(d) Molecular mass of polymers can be determined.

Concept of Osmosis and Osmotic Pressure

The experimental setup for demonstrating the osmosis experiment is shown in Fig. A thistle tube has a wide opening at one end. A piece of untreated cellophane is stretched and tied. The tube is partly filled with a concentrated solution of sucrose (a non-volatile solute). The thistle tube is immersed in a beaker of water.

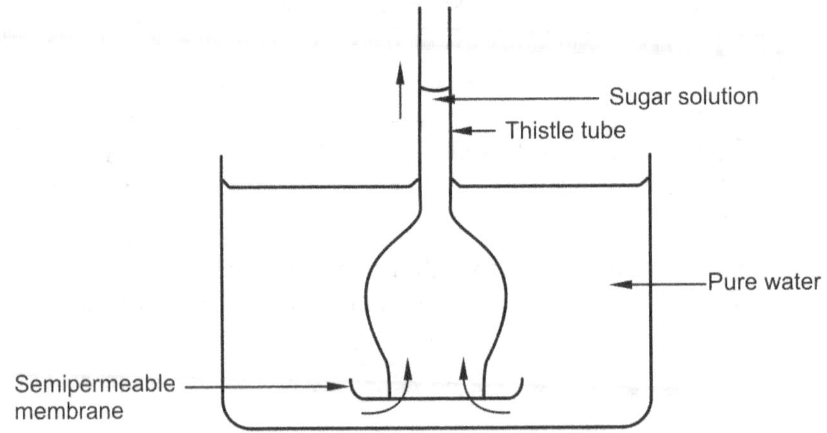

Fig. 4.11 Apparatus for demonstrating osmosis.

The diffusion of solvent molecules takes place in both directions. But number of water molecules that pass from beaker into sugar solution through semi-permeable membrane is more. Because of this the sugar solution is diluted and raises the vapour pressure to its original value. This process creates enough pressure to drive the sugar solution rise up in the tube. At one point, the rise of solution in tube stops, i.e., equilibrium is achieved.

At equilibrium

Hydrostatic pressure of the column of liquid = Flow of water (osmotic pressure) causing the water to pass through the membrane and enters the tube.

Since the V.P of solvent is higher than that of solute, water molecules diffuse.

Osmotic pressure is define as the hydrostatic pressure build up on solution, which just stops the osmosis of pure water into the solution, through a semi-permeable membrane also it can be defined as the external pressure applied to the solution in order to stop osmosis of solvent into solution separated by a semi permeable membrane.

Measurement of Osmotic Pressure

The osmotic pressure of a solution can be determined experimentally by various methods. It is not measured by observing the height that is attained in the thistle tube at equilibrium for following reason: The concentration of the final solution is not known because the concentration is continuously altered due to passage of water molecules. Direct measure of osmotic pressure remains difficult and inconvenient.

The apparatus used for this purpose is often referred to as osmometre

Berkely and Hartley's Osmometre Method

In this type, external pressure is applied on the solution just enough to prevent osmosis.

Construction: The osmometre is shown in Fig. A porcelain tube with copper ferrocyanide membrane deposited in its walls is enclosed in a metallic jacket. The tube is connected to a reservoir of pure solvent (water) at one end. A capillary tube is fixed at the other. Mechanical pressure can be applied on the solution with a piston connected through a pressure gauge.

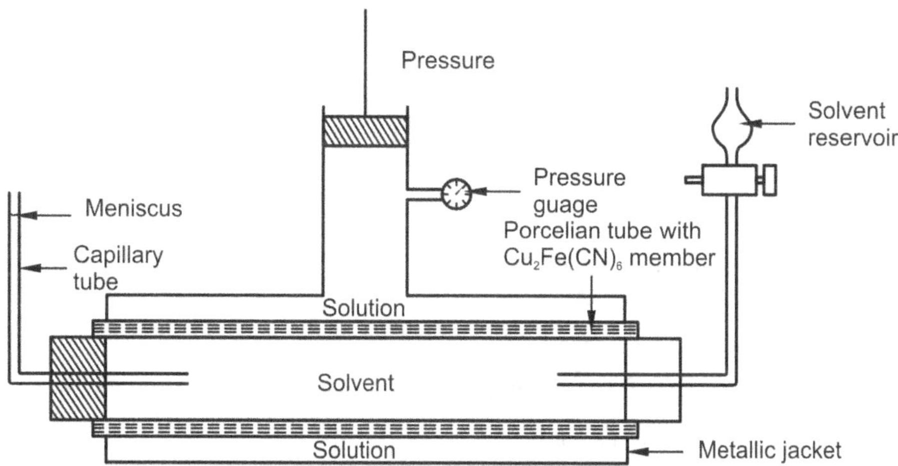

Fig. 4.12 Berkeley and Hartley's osmometre.

Procedure: The inner porcelain tube is filled with pure solvent and the jacket is filled with the solution whose osmotic-pressure is to be determined. The level of the solvent meniscus in the capillary tube will tend to move down as solvent flows into the solution across the membrane. Pressure is then applied through the piston so that the meniscus becomes stationary. It indicates that osmosis has been stopped and now the pressure recorded by the pressure gauge gives the osmotic pressure of solution.

Advantages: Berkeley and Hartley's method is fairly good and gives quick and accurate results. It can be used for determining high osmotic pressure. Since the external pressure balances the osmotic pressure, there is no strain left on the membranes and the danger of its bursting is limited.

Laws of Osmotic Pressure – Van't Hoff Equation

Dilute solutions of non electrolytes are found to obey the laws analogues to gas laws. For dilute solutions Van't Hoff showed that:

(a) The osmotic pressure of a solution at a given temperature is directly proportional to its concentration, i.e., $\pi \propto C$. It can also be written as $\pi \propto \left(\dfrac{1}{V}\right)$, where 'V' is the volume of the solution.

(b) The osmotic pressure of a solution of a given concentration is directly proportional to the absolute temperature

   i.e., $\qquad\qquad\qquad \pi \propto T$

Van't Hoff considered that the above equations can be totally represented as:

$$\pi V = n\,RT \qquad \text{Van't Hoff equation} \qquad \text{.....(4.10)}$$

π = osmotic pressure, KP_a

V = volume of the solution

n = number of kilogram moles of solute, K mol

R = ideal gas constant (= 8.3143 KJ/L mol. K)

T = absolute temperature, K

Osmotic pressures are high for example, 1 K mol of solute in 1 m^3 of solution (i.e., 1 mol in litre) gives a pressure at 300 K as:

$$\pi = 8.3143 \times 300$$

$$= 2490\ KP_a$$

The eq. 4.10 can also be represented as:

$$\pi = \frac{n}{V}\,RT = CRT$$

When the concentration is expressed in molality rather than molarity, the results obtained are comparatively nearer to experimental findings.

$$\pi = m\,RT \qquad \text{Morse equation}$$

$$m = \text{molality}$$

All the Van't Hoff equation and Morse equation are valid only for dilute solutions, if there is no dissociation and association of solute molecules.

Osmotic Pressure–Molecular Mass

The Van't Hoff and Morse equations may be used for calculating the molecular mass of solutes (particularly polymers such as proteins) from osmotic pressure, provided the solution is insufficiently dilute and ideal.

The Van't Hoff equation:

$$\pi = C\,R\,T$$

Replacing 'C' with C_g/M in above equation

$$\pi = \frac{C_g}{M}\,RT \qquad\qquad .....(4.11)$$

C_g = concentration of the solute, Kg/m^3 (or g/lt)

M = molecular mass of the polymer, (g/mol)

Rearranging the eq. 4.11, gives

$$\frac{\pi}{C_g} = \frac{RT}{M}$$

The quantity (C_g/M) is often a liner function of the concentration, C_g. This expression may be written as

$$\frac{\pi}{C_g} = \frac{RT}{M} + B\,C_g$$

where,

B is a constant for any particular solvent/solute system and depends on the degree of interaction between the solvent and solute molecules.

A plot of (C_g/M) against C_g, results in a straight line. The intercept is (RT/M). If the temperature at which the determination is carried out is known, it is possible to determine molecular mass.

4.5 Questions

1. Write the difference between Ideal and Real solutions with suitable examples.

2. What are colligative properties? Derive an expression for the determination of elevation of boiling point.

3. What are colligative properties? Derive an expression for the calculation of molecular weight of nonvolatile solute by freezing point depression method.

4. How do you express the pharmaceutical concentration of solution.

CHAPTER 5

SOLUTIONS OF ELECTROLYTES

5.1 Introduction

In 1887, the first satisfactory theory of ionic solutions was proposed by Arrhenius. The theory was based largely on studies of:

(i)   Electric conductance by kohlrausch

(ii)   Colligative properties by Van't Hoff

(iii) Chemical properties by Thomsen

Eg: Heat of Neutralisation

Arrhenius was able to bring the results of these diverse investigations into a broad generalisation known as the theory of electrolytic dissociation.

The theory was useful for describing weak electrolytes and it was soon found unsatisfactory for strong and moderately strong electrolytes. Accordingly many attempts were made to modify or replace Arrhenius's ideas with better ones and finally, in 1923, Debye and Huckel put forth a new theory. It is based on the principle that strong electrolytes are completely dissociated into ion in solutions of moderate concentration and the complete dissociation may be deviated due to interionic attractions.

Debye and Huckel expressed the deviations in terms of activities, activity coefficients and ionic strength's of electrolytic solutions. These quantities, which had been introduced earlier by Lewis, are discussed in this chapter together with the theory of interionic attraction. Other aspects of modern ionic theory and the relationships between electricity and chemical phenomena are considered in following chapters.

5.2 Properties of Solutions of Electrolytes

Electrolysis

Definition:

Under a potential of several volts, a direct electric current (dc) flows through an electrolytic cell (Fig. 5.1), when chemical reaction occurs. The process is known as electrolysis.

When a potential is applied, Fig. 5.1 electrons enter the cell from the battery or generator at the cathode. The electrons combine with positive ions or cations in the solution and hence the cations are reduced. The negative ions, or anions, carry electrons through the solution and discharge them at the anode and hence get oxidised. Reduction is the addition of electrons to a chemical species, and oxidation is removal of electrons from a species. The current in the solution constitutes flow of positive and negative ions towards the electrodes, whereas the current in a metallic conductor constitutes flow of free electrons migrating through a crystal lattice of fixed positive ions. Reduction occurs at the cathode where electrons are added to chemical species in solution. Oxidation occurs at the anode where electrons are removed from chemical species in solution.

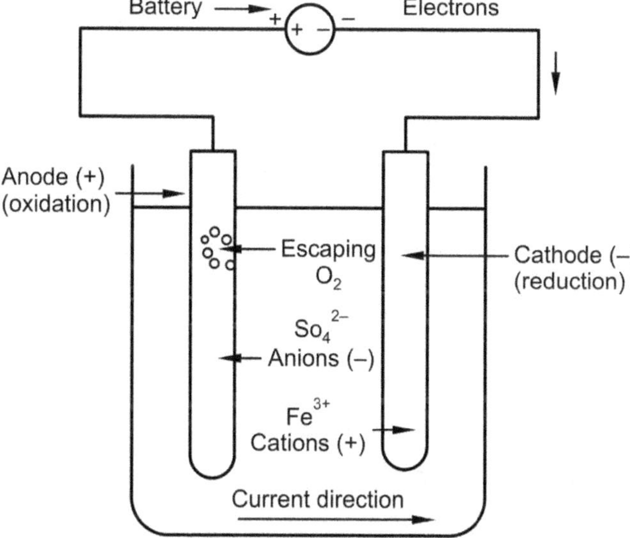

Fig. 5.1 Electrolysis in an Electrolytic cell.

For example, in the electrolysis of solution of ferric sulphate containing platinum electrodes,

Reaction at Cathode:

$$Fe^{3+} + e \rightarrow Fe^{2+}$$

Ferric ion   Ferrous ion

The sulphate ion is not easily oxidised and hence hydroxyl ions of water are converted into molecular oxygen, which escapes at the anode, and sulphuric acid is found in the solution at the electrode.

Reaction at Anode

$$OH^- \rightarrow \frac{1}{4} O_2 + \frac{1}{2} H_2O + e^-$$

Platinum electrodes are used here because they do not pass into solution to any extent. When attackable metals, such as Copper or Zinc, are used as the anode, their atoms tend to lose electrons, and the metal passes into solution as the positively charged ion.

Transference Numbers

The fraction of total current carried by the cations or by the anions is known as transport or transference number t_+ or t_-:

$$t_+ = \frac{\text{Current carried by cations}}{\text{Total current}}$$

$$t_- = \frac{\text{Current carried by Anions}}{\text{Total current}}$$

The sum of two transference numbers is equal to unity

$$t_+ + t_- = 1$$

In the electrolysis, flow of electrons through the solution from right to left in Fig. 5.1 is accomplished by the movement of cations to the right as well as anions to the left.

The transference numbers are related to the velocities of the ions, the faster-moving ion carrying the greater fraction of current.

For example, transference number of sodium ion in a 0.10M solution of NaCl is 0.385 and Lithium ion in a 0.10M solution of LiCl has a transference number of 0.317.

Electrical Units

According to Ohm's law, the strength of an electric current (I) flowing through a metallic conductor is related to the difference in applied voltage or potential (E) and the resistance (R).

$$I = \frac{E}{R}$$

The current strength I is the rate of flow of current or quantity Q of electricity flowing per unit time

$$I = \frac{Q}{T}$$

Quantity of electric charge,   Q = current,   I × Time, t

Q is expressed in columb,   C in amperes,   and   E in volts

5.3 Electrolytic Conductance

The ability of metals to conduct an electric current results from the mobility of electrons in the metals. This type of conductivity is called "metallic conductance". On the other hand, various chemical compounds such as acids, bases and salt conduct electricity by virtue of ions present or formed rather than by electrons. This is called "electrolytic conductance" and the conducting compounds are called electrolytes.

The electrolytic conductivity of a solution of electrolyte is the reciprocal of the resistance of the solution

$$\therefore \qquad\qquad C = \frac{1}{R} \qquad\qquad\qquad .....(5.1)$$

C = Conductor,   R = Resistance

R is given by

$$R = \rho \frac{l}{A}$$

ρ = resistance between opposite face of a 1 cm cube of a conductor i.e., specific resistance

l = length of conductor, cm

A   = cross sectional area of conductor, cm^2

Specific conductance, K is the reciprocal of specific resistance

$$K = \frac{1}{\rho}$$

The relationship between K and C or R is given by

$$K = C.\frac{l}{A} = \frac{1}{R}.\frac{l}{A} \qquad \qquad \dots\dots(5.2)$$

Units : mhos

Measuring the Electrolytic Conductance of Solutions

The wheatstone bridge for measuring the conductance of a solution is shown in Fig. 5.2. The solution of unknown resistance R_x is placed in the cell and connected in the circuit. The contact point is moved along the slide wire bc until at same point, say d, no current from the source of alternating current (oscillator) flows through the detector. When the bridge is balanced, the potential at a is equal to that at d, the sound in the earphones or the oscillating pattern on the oscilloscope is at a minimum, and the resistance R_3, R_1 and R_2 are R.ad. In the balanced state, the resistance of solution R_x is obtained from the equation

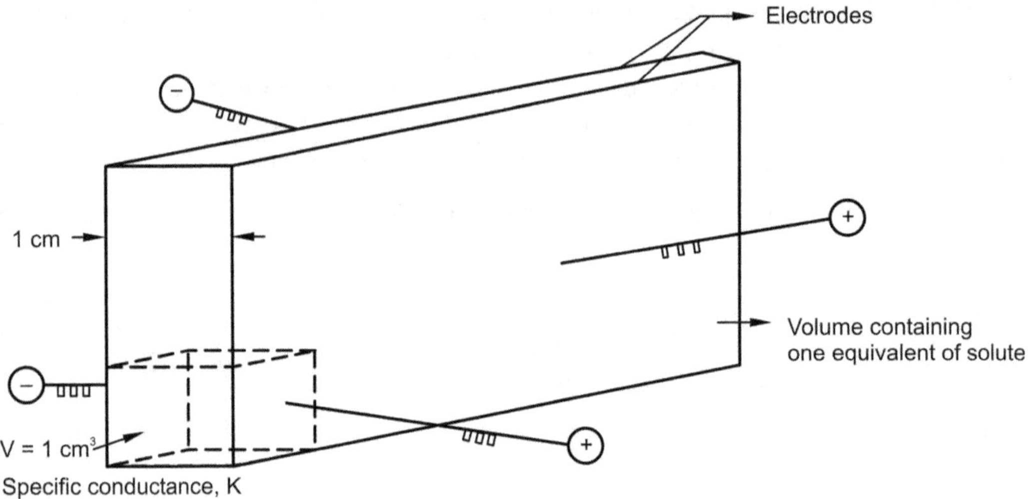

Fig. 5.2 Relationship between specific conductance and equivalent conductance.

$$R_x = R_s \frac{R_1}{R_2}$$

Since to measure conductivity is actually to measure electrical resistance, "C" can be easily calculated

5.4 Equivalent Conductance

Equivalent conductance Λ is defined as the conductance of a solution of sufficient volume to contain 1 gm equivalent of the solute when measured in a cell in which the electrodes are spaced 1cm apart.

Since specific conductance measures the current carrying capacity of all ions in a unit volume of solution which varies with concentration to study the dissociation of molecules into ions, equivalent conductance is more useful than specific conductance, independent of concentration of electrolyte.

Equivalent conductance is given by

$$\Lambda_c = KV_e$$

K = Specific conductance

V_e = Volume in millilitres

$$\Lambda_c = KV_e = \frac{1000K}{C} \text{ m ho cm}^2/\text{eq}$$

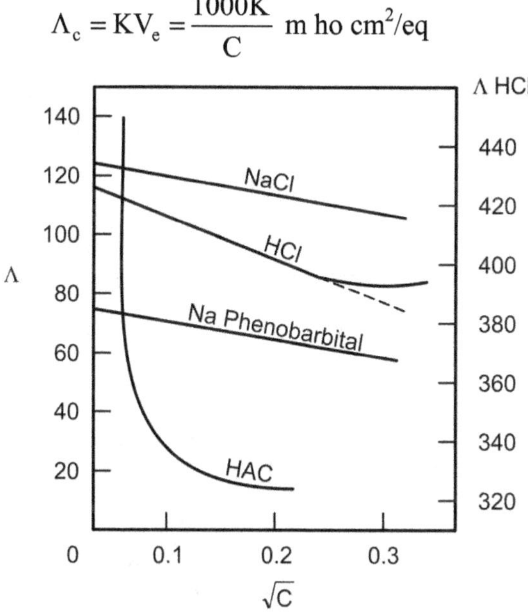

Fig. 5.3 Equivalent conductance of strong and weak Electrolytes.

Equivalent Conductance of Strong and Weak Electrolytes

Electrolytes are broadly classified as strong and weak electrolytes. The former includes solutions of strong acids, strong base and most salts; the latter includes weak acid and bases, primarily organic acids, amine and a few salts. The criterion for this is extent of "ionisation".

The equivalent conductances of some electrolytes at different concentrations are given in Table 5.2 and Fig. 5.3.

As the solution of strong electrolyte is diluted, the specific conductance K decreases because the number of ions per unit volume of solution is reduced and equivalent conductance of Λ_c a solution of a strong electrolyte increases on dilution. The equivalent conductance of a weak electrolyte also increases on dilution, but not as rapidly as first.

Kohlrausch was one of the investigators, to find that the equivalent conductance was a linear function of the square root of the concentration for strong electrolytes in dilute solution, as illustrated in Fig. 5.3. The expression for Λ at a concentration "C" is

$$\Lambda_c = \Lambda_0 - b\sqrt{c} \qquad .....(5.4)$$

$\Lambda_0 =$ Intercept on vertical axis, known as equivalent conductance at infinite dilution

b = slope of line for strong electrolytes shown in Figure.

For example, the value of Λ_0 for acetic acid may be calculated as

$$\Lambda_0\,(CH_3COOH) = \Lambda_0\,(HCl) + \Lambda_0\,(CH_3OONa) - \Lambda_0\,(NaCl)$$

which is equivalent to

$$C_0(H^+) + Co\,(CH_3COO^-) = CO(H^+) + Co(Cl^-) + Co(Na^+) + Co\,(CH_3COO^-)$$
$$- \quad Co(Na^+) - Co\,(Cl^-)$$

The values of NaCl, HCl, CH_3 COOH are determined by extrapolation and substitution of these gives a value of 3906 for Λ_0 (Table 5.2).

At infinite dilution, Λ_0 is the sum of cations equivalent conductance of cations C_c^o and the anions C_a^o,

$$\Lambda_0 = C_c^o + C_a^o$$

Colligative Properties of Electrolytic Solutions and Concentrated Solutions of Non-electrolytes

When a non-volatile solute is dissolved in a solvent, certain properties of the resultant solution are largely independent of the nature of the solute and are determined by the concentration of solute particles. These properties are called "Colligative properties".

Osmotic pressure is one of the colligative properties. According to Van't Hoff, the osmotic pressure of a dilute solution of non-electrolyte is expressed by following equation

$$\pi = RTC \qquad .....(5.5)$$

$\pi =$ Osmotic pressure of solution, P_0

R = Gas constant, J/mol. K

T = Absolute temperature, K

C = Concentration of solute, moles/ litre

However solutions of strong electrolytes such as salt gave osmotic pressure twice or thrice as large as would be expected based on eq. 5.5. Hence a correction factor (i) is introduced in eq. 5.5 for electrolytes

$$\pi = i\,CRT$$

The Vant Hoff factor (i) is equal to number of ions produced on dissociation of one molecule as the solution is diluted.

i, may be expressed as

$$i = \frac{\text{Observed colligative property}}{\text{Colligative property expected if dissociation does not occur}} \qquad .....(5.6)$$

In terms of osmotic pressure

$$i = \frac{\pi}{\pi_0} = \frac{\text{Osmotic pressure of electrolyte}}{\text{Osmotic pressure if ionization does not occur}}$$

For example, if NaCl is completely ionised, one mole of NaCl gives 2 moles of ions (Na^+ and Cl^-). Therefore

$$i = \frac{\pi}{\pi_0} = 2$$

The i factor is plotted against the molal concentration of electrolyte and non-electrolytes, as shown in Fig. 5.4.

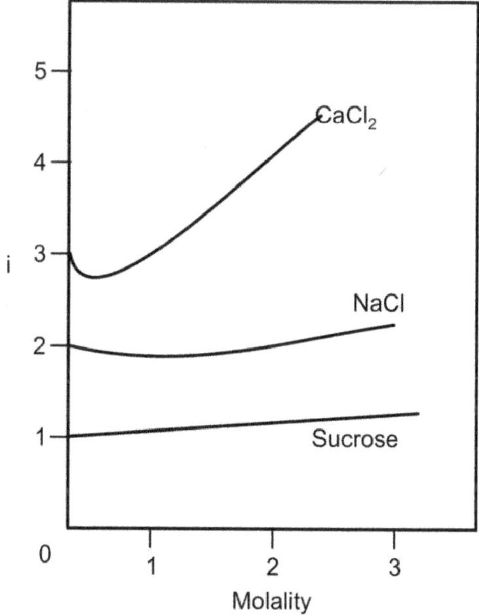

Fig. 5.4 Van't Hoff i factor of representative compounds.

5.5 Faraday's Laws of Electrolysis

Electrolysis is considered as chemical decomposition of an electrolyte. Faradays laws describe the quantitative relationship between the quantity of electric current used and amount of chemical reaction brought about by the current.

Faraday's First law

It states that the amount of chemical decomposition produced is proportional to the quantity of electricity flows through an electrolyte.

$$W \propto It$$

$$W = Itz$$

W = Weight of substance deposited

I = Current strength, A

T = Time, s

Z = Electrochemical equivalent, a constant

when $I = 1$, $t = 1$,   then $W = Z$

Electrochemical equivalent is defined as the amount of a substance deposited by 1 ampere of current passing for one second.

The equivalent weight of any substance is same i.e., one mole. A mole of any substance contains 6.02×10^{23} atoms or molecules. In other words, one mole of atoms requires a mole of electrons i.e., 6.02×10^{23} to deposit as metal.

According to first law chemical decomposition is not influenced by the electrodes, (or) by the cell and also independent of temperature.

Faraday's Second Law

It states that when the same quantity of electricity is passed through different electrolytes, the amount of product deposited is proportional to their chemical equivalent.

Consider Fig. 5.5 for illustrating the second law of Faraday. Same quantity of electricity is passed through three cell, containing solutions of dil. H_2SO_4, $CuSO_4$ and Ag NO_3 respectively. The amounts of H_2, Cu and Ag liberated at the cathodes are estimated.

When one Coloumb of electricity is passed, the amounts deposited are:

Hydrogen = 0.00001036 g

Copper = 0.0003292 g

Silver = 0.001118 g

The quantity of current needed to deposit the equivalent weight will be

$$\text{Hydrogen} \quad = \quad \frac{1}{0.00001036} \quad = 96{,}525 \text{ Coloumb}$$

$$\text{Copper} \quad = \quad \frac{31.78}{0.0003292} \quad = 96{,}537 \text{ Coloumb}$$

$$\text{Silver} \quad = \quad \frac{107.88}{0.00118} \quad = 96{,}494 \text{ Coloumb}$$

The chemical equivalents of H, Cu, Ag are 1, 31.78, 107.88. The proportionalities constant can be obtained as

$$H_2 = 1 \times 0.00001036 \qquad = 0.00001036 \text{ g}$$
$$Cu = 31.78 \times 0.00001036 \qquad = 0.0003292 \text{ g}$$
$$Ag = 107.88 \times 0.00001036 \qquad = 0.001118 \text{ g}$$

It follows that electrochemical equivalents are proportional to the chemical equivalents.

The current in Coloumbs obtained may be rounded to 96,500 and it is known as Faraday, denoted by F. One Faraday = 96, 500 coloumb.

In SI units, $\quad F = 9.6493 \times 10^7 \text{ C/keg}$

Applications

1. Faraday's laws can be used to compute the charge of an electron.

2. Second law of electrolysis is utilised in the determination of equivalent weights of metals.

5.6 Arrhenius's Theory of Electrolytic Dissociation

The Swedish chemist Svante Arrhenius prepared a doctoral on the properties of electrolytes at the University of Uppsala in Sweden. According to Arrhenius, when electrolytes are dissolved in water, the solute exists in the form of ions in the solution, as seen in the following equations:

$$Na^+Cl^- + H_2O \quad \longrightarrow \quad Na^+ + Cl^- + H_2O \qquad \dots\dots(i)$$

[Ionic compound] $\qquad\qquad$ [Strong Electrolyte] $\quad$ Ionic

$$HCl + H_2O \quad \longrightarrow \quad H_3O^+ + Cl^- \qquad \dots\dots(ii)$$

[Covalent compound] $\qquad\qquad$ [Strong electrolyte] $\quad$ covalent

$$CH_3COOH + H_2O \quad \rightleftharpoons \quad H_3O^+ + CH_3COO^- \qquad \dots\dots(iii)$$

[Covalent compound] $\qquad\qquad$ [Weak electrolyte] $\quad$ covalent

The solid form of sodium chloride is marked with plus and minus signs in eq. (i) to indicate that sodium chloride exists as ions even in the crystalline state. If electrode are connected to a source of current and are placed in a mass of fused NaCl, the molten compound will conduct the electric current because the crystal lattice of the pure salt consists of ions. The addition of water to the solid dissolves the crystal and separates the ions in the solution.

HCl exists essentially as neutral molecules rather than ions in the pure form and does not conduct electricity. When it reacts with H_2O, it ionizes according to the reaction. H_3O^+ is the hydrogen ion in water known as hydronium or oxonium ion. In addition to H_3O^+, other hydrated species of the proton probably exist in solution. Eg. H_2SO_4, HNO_3.

Acetic acid is a weak electrolyte in which molecules and ions are in equilibrium. It is indicated by oppositely directed arrows.

Inorganic acids : Boric acid   Inorganic bases : NH_4OH

Inorganic bases : $HgCl_2$ and HgI

Complex ions : $Hg(NH_3)_2^+$

Postulates

1. When electrolytes are dissolved in water, they undergo spontaneous dissociation to form oppositely charged ions.
2. The total no. of positively charged ions is equal to totals no. of negatively charged ions.
3. In solution, cation and anions are responsible for conducting electric current. This is similar to Faraday's proposal.
4. Arrhenius considered that strong electrolytes are completely dissociated whereas weak electrolyte, dissociate to a low extent, which is indicated by the equilibrium condition.

Limitation

1. It does not explain the role of solvent in process of dissociation
2. It does not consider the electrostatic force of attraction between the ions.
3. This theory does not explain the process of ionisation

Classification of Substances

Arrhenius classified all substances into two classes.

(i)   Electrolytes

(ii) Non-electrolytes

I Electrolytes

Substances which have capacity to carry current or which produce ions in solutions when dissolved in water.

These are further classified based on extent of ionisation.

1. Strong electrolytes
2. Weak electrolytes

1. *Strong electrolytes:* Substance which completely dissociate into ions in solution of moderate concentration

   Ionic – $NaCl$, KNO_3, $NaOH$, Covalent : HCl, H_2SO_4, HNO_3

2. *Weak electrolytes:* These are substance which dissociate to a low degree and conduct current feebly in aqueous solution.

   e.g.: Organic acids : Acetic acid, Citric acid

   e.g.: Organic bases : Methyl amine and Aniline

II Non-Electrolytes

These are substances which contain molecules i.e. which do not dissociate into ions and cannot carry current are called non-electrolytes.

Eg: Sucrose, Urea and Glycerin

Drugs and Ionization

Some drugs, such as anionic and cationic antibacterial and antiprotozoal agents are more active when in the ionic state. Other compounds, such as hydroxybenzene, esters and many general anaesthetics, bring about their biologic effects as non electrolytes. Still other compounds, such as sulphonamides are thought to exert their drug action both as anions and a neural molecules.

Degree of Dissociation

When Arhenius introduced his theory of ionisation, he proposed that the degree of ionisation, α, of an electrolyte is measured by the ratio.

$$\alpha = \Lambda_c / \Lambda_o \qquad\qquad .....(5.8)$$

The ratio is known as "Conductance ratio"

Λ_c = Equivalent conductance of an electrolyte at any specified concentration C.

Λ_o = Equivalent conductance at infinite dilution

He recognised that equivalent conductance at infinite dilution, Λ_o was a measure of the complete dissociation of the solute into its ions and that Λ_c represented the number of solute particles present as ions at a concentration.

The Van't Hoff factor, i can be connected with the degree of dissociation, α as

$$i = 1 + \alpha\,(v - 1)$$

$$\alpha = \frac{i - 1}{v - 1}$$

γ = no.of ions into which the electrolyte dissociate.

$$i = 1 + \alpha\,(v - 1)$$

$$\because T_f = i\,K_f\,m$$

i can be calculated by

$$i = \frac{\Delta T_f}{K_f m} \qquad\qquad .....(5.9)$$

ΔT_f = Freezing point depression, K

K_f = Molar depression constant, °C. Kg/mol

m = Concentration of solute, molal.

5.7 Theory of Strong Electrolytes

The Arrhenius theory explains why solutions of electrolytes conduct electricity, and why they exhibit enhanced colligative properties. The theory is satisfactory for solutions of weak electrolytes.

In case of strong electrolytes:

(i) It does not explain the failure of strong electrolytes to follow the law of mass action as applied to ionisation

(ii) Discrepancies exist between the α calculated from i, and the conductivity ratio for strong electrolyte solutions having concentrations greater than 0.5 M.

According to the early ionic theory, the degree of dissociation of NH_4Cl, a strong electrolyte, was calculated in the same manner as that of weak electrolyte. The Arrhenius theory is now accepted for describing the behaviour only of weak electrolytes. The α of weak electrolytes can be calculated from conductance ratio.

The deficiencies of Arrhenius theory can be explained by the following observations.

1. In the molten state, strong electrolytes are excellent conductors of electricity. This suggests that these materials are already ionised in the crystalline state. Further support is given by x-ray studies of crystals.

2. Arrhenius neglected the fact that ions in solution, being oppositely charged, tend to associate through electrostatic attraction. In solutions of weak electrolytes, the number of ions is not large and it is not surprising that electrostatic attractions do not cause appreciable deviations from theory.

Activity and Activity Coefficients

As a solution become more concentrated, due to increased electrostatic attractions, the concentration of an ion become less efficient as a measure of its net effectiveness. A more efficient measure of the physical or chemical effectiveness of an ion is known as its "Activity".

At infinite dilution, in which the ions are so widely separated that they do not interact with one another, the activity a of an ion is equal to its concentration, expressed as molality or molarity. It is written as

$$a = m \text{ (or)}$$

$$\frac{a}{m} = 1$$

as the concentration of the solution is increased, the ratio becomes less than unity. This ratio is known as the practical activity coefficient, r_m on the molal scale, and the formula is written as

$$\frac{a}{m} = r_m$$

$$a = r_m \, m \qquad\qquad\qquad .....(5.10)$$

On the molarity scale, another practical activity co-efficient, r_c is defined as

$$a = r_c \, C$$

On the mole fraction scale, a rational activity co-efficient is defined as

$$a = r_x \, X$$

The three coefficients usually decrease and assume different values as the concentration is increased.

The activity of an electrolyte is defined by its mean ionic activity, which is given by the relation.

$$a_{\pm} = (a_+^{\,m} \, a_-^{\,n})^{1/(m+n)}$$

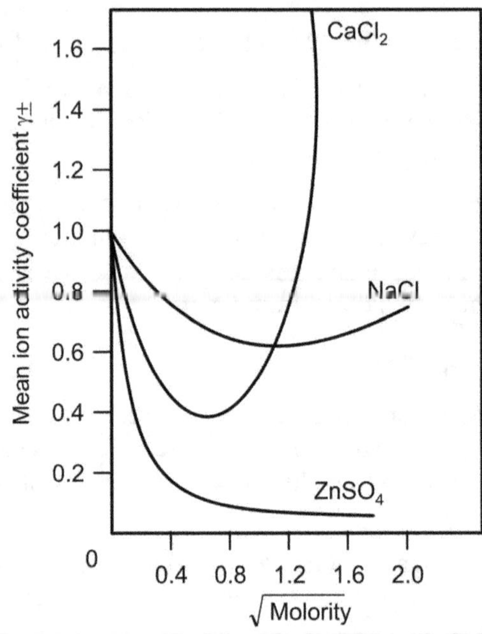

Fig. 5.5 Mean ionic activity coefficients of representative electrolytes plotted against the square root of concentrations.

It is possible to obtain the mean ionic activity co-efficient, $\gamma_\pm$ of an electrolyte by several experimental methods. Such as distribution co-efficient studies, electro motive force measurements, colligative property methods and solubility determination.

The mean ionic activity co-efficient of a number of strong electrolytes are given in Table 5.3 and the mean value of NaCl, $CaCl_2$, $ZnSO_4$ are plotted in Figure 4.5 against the activity square root of the molality.

Activity of the Solvent

When a solution is made infinitely dilute, it can be considered to consist of essentially of pure solvent. Therefore $X_1 \cong 1$, and the solvent behaves ideally in conformity with Raoult's Law, under this condition, the mole fraction can be set equal to the activity of the solvent, or

$$a = X_1 = 1$$

As the solution become more concentrated, the ratio is given by rational activity co-efficient.

$$\frac{a}{X_1} = r_x$$

$$a = r_x X_1 \qquad\qquad .....(5.11)$$

Activity is also given by

$$a_1 = p_1/p^o$$

p_1 = Vapour pressure of solvent in solution

p^o = Vapour pressure of pure solvent

Debye-Huckel Theory

Debye-Huckel theory is based upon the principles that strong electrolytes are completely ionized and ions experience attraction with neighbouring ions.

The equation relates the activity co-efficient of a particular ion or mean ionic activity coefficient of an electrolyte to the valence of the ions, ionic strength of the solution and the characteristic of solvent.

$$\log \gamma_i = - AZ_i^2 \sqrt{\mu} \qquad \text{(ionic strength up to 0.2)} \qquad ..... (5.12)$$

γ_i = Activity coefficient of ion

Z_i = Valence of the ion

μ = ionic strength of all ions

A = factor

For water $A = 0.51$

For ionic strength less than 0.02 (dilute solution)

$$\log \gamma_\pm = -AZ_{+} z_{-} \sqrt{\mu}$$

The above equation is for binary electrolytes consisting of ions in with valences of Z_{+} and Z_{-}.

Debye Huckel a theory can be extended to more concentrated solutions (about 0.1) by

$$\log r_\pm = \frac{- A_z + z - \sqrt{\mu}}{1 + a_i B\sqrt{\mu}}$$

where a_i is the mean distance of approach of ions and is called mean effective ionic diameter or ion size parameter

Since for water $B = 0.33 \times 10^8$ at 25°

for most electrolytes $a_i = 3$ to 4×10^{-8}

the product of a_i and B gives unity. Hence the equation becomes

$$\log r_\pm = \frac{A_z + z - \sqrt{\mu}}{1 + \sqrt{\mu}}$$

When ionic strength of the solution becomes high (approximately 0.3-0.5), these equations become inadequate and a linear term in μ is added. Hence eq become

$$\log r_{\pm} = \frac{A_z + z - \sqrt{\mu}}{1 + \sqrt{\mu}} + C\mu$$

Values of A and B for water are shown in Table 6.4.

Co-efficient for Expressing Colligative Properties L-Value

The Van't Hoff expression is

$$\Delta T_f = i\, K_f m$$

It is suitable for computing the colligative properties of non electrolytes, weak electrolytes and strong electrolytes.

It can be modified slightly for convenience in dilute solutions by substituting molar concentration c and by writing K_f as L, so that

$$\Delta T_f = Lc$$

L varies with the concentration of solution. At a concentration of drug that is isotonic with body fluids, $L = iKf$ is given as L is 0.

L value for

    Non-electrolytes is 1.9

    Weak electrolytes is 2.0

    Uni-valent electrolytes is 3.4

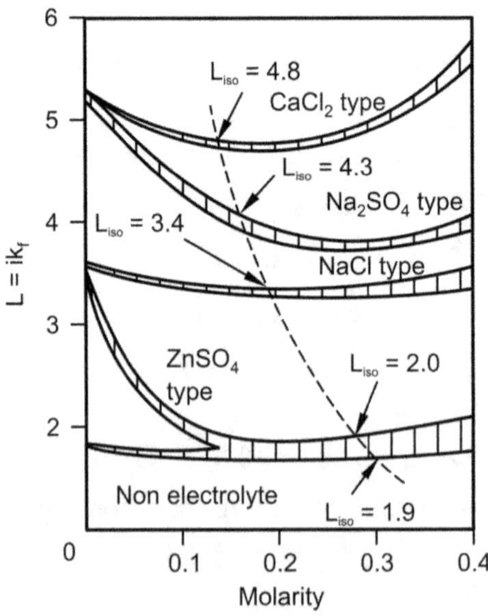

Fig. 5.6 Liso values of various ionic classes

A plot of iK_f against the concentration of some drug is presented in Fig. 5.6.

In this, each curve is represented by band to show the variability of L-values within each ionic class.

Osmotic Coefficient

Different method of correcting deviations of electrolytes from ideal colligative behaviour has been suggested. One of these is based on the fact that as the solution becomes more dilute, i, approaches v, the number of ions into which an electrolyte dissociate.

At infinite dilute dilution, $i = v$ or

$$i/v = 1$$

The ratio i/v is designated as g and is known as the practical osmotic coefficient

Osmotic coefficient, g, for electrolytes and nonelectrolytes are plotted against ionic concentration, vm in Fig. 5.7

Because $g = i/v$ or $i = gv$, the cryoscopic equation becomes

$$i = \frac{\Delta Tf}{Kf_m}$$

$$\Delta Tf = gvK_f m$$

The molar osmotic co-efficients of some salts are listed in Table.

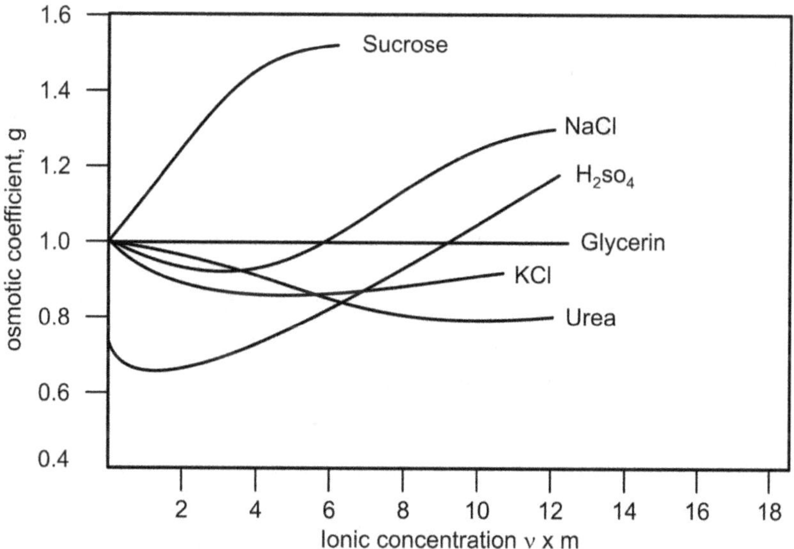

Fig. 5.7 Osmotic coefficient 'g' for some common solutes

Osmolality

A solution has an osmolol concentration of one when it contain, 1 osmol of solute/kg of water. A solution has an osmolality of n when it contains n osmol/kg of water. Osmolality reflect a weight to weight relationship between the solute and the solvent.

For electrolytes like NaCl, 1 osmol is approximately 0.5 mol of NaCl. Thus, it follows that 1 osmolal solution of NaCl essentially is equivalent to a 0.5 molal solution.

As in molal solutions, osmolar solutions usually are employed where quantitative precision is required, as in the measurement of physical and chemical properties of solution. The advantage of the w/w relationship is that concentration of the system is not influenced by temperature.

For an electrolyte that dissociates into ions in a dilute solution, osmolality can be calculated from:

$$\text{Milli osmolality} = i\text{-}mm$$

i = No.of ions formed per molecule

mm = millimolar concentration

Osmolarity is the no. of osmoles per litre of solution and osmality is the no. of osmoles per kilogram of solvent.

Osmolarity can be calculated from osmolality by

$$\text{Osmolarity} = \text{Measured osmolarity} \times \text{solution density in g/ms}$$

$$- \text{Anhydrous solute concentration. in g/ml}$$

Osmolality is converted into osmolarity by

$$\text{MOSm/litre solution} = \text{MOSm/(kg } H_2O) \times [\, d_1^0 \, (1 - 0.001 \, \overline{V}_2^o]$$

$d_1{}^\circ$ = Density of solvent

$\overline{V}_2{}^\circ$ = Partial molar volume of solute at infinite dilution

5.8 Questions

1. Explain the Arrhenius theory of electrolytic dissociation. Give its limitations.

2. What is electrolytic conductance and how will you measure the electrolytic conductance of solutions.

3. Describe Faraday's laws of electrolysis.

4. Discuss "Debye-Huckel Theory" under theory of strong electrolytes.

CHAPTER 6

IONIC EQUILIBRIA

6.1 Introduction

1. ***Earlier concept of acid and base:*** An acid may be defined as any substance which has a sour taste and its aqueous solution turns blue litmus to red.

   A base may be defined as any substance which has a bitter taste and its aqueous solution turns red litmus to blue

   Limitations: This concept could not explain the behaviour of all acids and bases.

Theory of Acid and Base

2. ***Arrhenius concept:*** According to Arrhenius, an acid may be defined as any hydrogen containing compound which gives H^+ ions in aqueous solution and a base may be defined as a substance containing hydroxy groups or groups capable of providing hydroxide ions (OH^-) in aqueous solution.

131

For example in following equations,

$$HCl \underset{}{\overset{H_2O}{\rightleftharpoons}} H^+ + Cl^-$$

$$NaOH \underset{}{\overset{H_2O}{\rightleftharpoons}} Na^+ + OH^-$$

HCl is an acid and NaOH is a base.

According to Arrhenius, neutralisation process can be represented by a reaction involving combination of H^+ and OH^- ions to form water.

$$H^+ + OH^- \rightarrow H_2O$$

Limitations

(a) The definitions of acid and base are only in terms of aqueous solutions and not in terms of substance.

(b) This theory not able to explain acidic and basic properties of substances in non-aqueous solvents. E.g., $NH_4 NO_3$ in NH_3^+ acts as an acid, though it does not give H^+ ions.

(c) The neutralisation of acid and base in absence of solvent could not be explained by the theory. Many organic substances and NH_3 which do not have OH^- ions at all are actually known to show basic characteristics.

(d) It cannot explain the acidic character of certain salts such as $AlCl_3$ in aqueous solution.

3. ***Bron sted-Lowry concept (proton-donor concept):*** According to this theory an acid may be defined as any hydrogen containing material that is capable of donating a proton H^+ to any other substance. A base may be defined as any substance that can accept a proton from any other substance, in short an acid is a proton donor and a base is a proton acceptor.

Some examples of acids are

$$HCL \rightleftharpoons H^+ + Cl^-$$

$$CH_3COOH \rightleftharpoons H^+ + CH_3 COO^-$$

$$H SO_4^- \rightleftharpoons H^+ + SO_4^{2-}$$

Some examples of bases are

$$OH^- + H^+ \rightleftharpoons H_2O$$

$$H_2O + H^+ \rightleftharpoons H_3O^+$$

$$SO_4^{2-} + H^+ \rightleftharpoons H SO_4^-$$

Conjugate Acid-base pairs: For example in a reaction.

$$\underset{\underset{1}{Acid}}{HCl} + \underset{\underset{2}{Base}}{H_2O} \rightleftharpoons \underset{\underset{2}{Acid}}{H_3O^+} + \underset{\underset{1}{Base}}{Cl^-}$$

In this reaction, HCl donates a proton to H_2O so it is an acid and water accepts a proton from HCl so it is a base. In the reverse reaction H_3O^+ ion donates a proton to Cl^- ion, so H_3O^+ is an acid, Cl^- ion accepts a proton form H_3O^+, so it is a base. The acid-base pairs, the members of which can be formed from each other mutually by the gain or loss of proton are called conjugate acid-base pairs.

In the above reaction, HCl is acid and it's conjugate base Cl^- as base and if H_2O is designated as base$_2$ and its conjugate acid H_3O^+ as acid$_2$.

Some examples

$$H_2SO_4 + H_2O \rightleftharpoons H_3O^+ + HSO_4^-$$

$$CH_3COOH + H_2O \rightleftharpoons H_3O^+ + CH_3COO^-$$

water is having dual character because it can accept a proton or donate. This can be illustrated in

$$H_2O + HCl \rightleftharpoons H_3O^+ + Cl^-$$

$$H_2O + NH_3 \rightleftharpoons NH_4^+ + OH^-$$

In the first reaction H_2O accepts a proton from HCl to form H_3O^+ so it acts as base. In second reaction H_2O donates a proton to NH_3 and forms OH^- ion so it acts as an acid.

Any substance which can donate as well as accepts a proton is termed as amphoteric or amphiprotic.

According to definition a strong acid is one which readily donates its proton to a base, so the conjugate base of such as acid must be weak. General rule is strong acids have weak conjugate bases and strong bases have weak conjugate acids.

Limitations

(i)   According to this theory, all acids are protonic in nature, yet there are many which are not.

(ii)   A large number of acid-base reactions are known in which no proton transfer can takes place. E.g.,

$$\underset{\underset{1}{Acid}}{SO_2} + \underset{\underset{2}{Base}}{SO_2} \rightleftharpoons \underset{\underset{2}{Base}}{SO_2^{2+}} + \underset{\underset{1}{Base}}{SO_3^{2-}}$$

4. ***Lewis concept (Electron donor-acceptor system)*** : According to Lewis, an acid may be defined as any species that can accept an electron pair to form a coordinate bond and a base may be defined as any species that can donate an electron pair to the formation of a coordinate bond. Thus in lewis system, an acid is an electron pair acceptor and a base is an electron pair donor. According to this theory, the process of neutralisation is the formation of a coordinate bond between an acid and a base.

$$H^+ + :NH_3 \longrightarrow H \longleftarrow NH_3$$
$$\text{Adduct}$$

In the above reaction proton (H^+) accepts one electron pair from : NH_3 molecule and is therefore an acid where as NH_3 molecule which donates an electron pair is a base. The adduct is NH_4^+ ion.

Another example is

$$BF_3 + : NH_3 \longrightarrow BF_3 \leftarrow NH_3$$

Here BF_3 accepts one lone pair of electrons and is therefore a lewis acid while NH_3 donates 1 lone pair of electrons and is therefore a lewis base.

Some examples of lewis acid are H^+, NH_4^+, Na^+, K^+, Cu^{+2}, Al^{3+} etc

Some examples of lewis base are NH_3, H_2O, OH^-, Cl^-, CN^-, S^{-2} etc

Limitations

(i)   Since the strength of Lewis acids and bases is found to depend on type of reaction, it is not possible to arrange them in any order of their relative strength.

(ii) As Lewis acid-base reactions involve electrons, they are expected to be very fast reactions but there are many lewis acid-base reactions which are slow.

5. ***Acid base equilibria***

The ionisation or protcolysis of a weak electrolyte, acetic acid in water can be written in Bronsted. Lowry manner as

$$\underset{\text{Acid}_1}{HAC} + \underset{\text{Base}_2}{H_2O} \rightleftharpoons \underset{\text{Acid}_2}{H_3O^+} + \underset{\text{Base}_1}{AC^-}$$

According to the law of mass action, the velocity or rate of the forward reaction, R_f is proportional to the concentration of the reactants.

$$R_f = K_1 \times [HAC]^1 \times [H_2O]^1 \qquad .....(6.1)$$

The speed of the reaction is usually expressed in terms of the decrease in the concentration of either the reactants per unit time.

$$R_r = K_2 \times [H_3O^+]^1 \times [AC^-]^1 \qquad \ldots..(6.2)$$

R_r is reformation of un-ionized acetic acid. Because only 1 mole of each constituent appears in the reaction, each term is raised to the first power and the exponents need not appear in subsequent expressions for dissociation of acetic acid and similar acids and bases. The symbols K_1 and K_2 are proportionality constants commonly known as specific reaction rates for forward and reverse reactions respectively and the brackets indicate concentrations.

6. *Ionization of weak acids*

According to concept of equilibrium the rate of the forward reactions decreases with time as acetic acid is depleted where as the rate of reverse reaction begins at zero and increases as larger quantities of hydrogen ions and acetate ions are formed. When 2 rates are equal i.e.,

$$R_f = R_r \qquad \ldots..(6.3)$$

The concentration of products and reactants are not equal at equilibrium, the speeds of forward and reverse reactions are same. Based on eq. 6.3, equation we can write.

$$K_1 \times [HAC] \times [H_2O] = K2 \times [H_3O^+] \times [AC^-] \qquad \ldots..(6.4)$$

$$K = \frac{K_1}{K_2} = \frac{[H_3O^+][AC^-]}{[HAC][H_2O]} \qquad \ldots..(6.5)$$

In dilute solutions of acetic acid, water is in sufficient excess to be regarded as constant at about 55.3 moles/lt. It is thus combined with K_1/K_2 to yield a new constant K_a, the ionization constant or dissociation constant of acetic acid.

$$K_a = 55.3 \, K = \frac{[H_3O^+][AC^-]}{[HAC]} \qquad \ldots..(6.6)$$

This equation is equilibrium expression for dissociation of acetic acid.

An equilibria involving charged as well as uncharged acids, Bronsted-Lowry nomenclature, the term ionisation constant K_a is replaced by acidity constant. Smimilarly for charged, uncharged bases the term basicity constant is used for K_b.

The acidity constant for uncharged weak acid HB can be expressed by

$$HB + H_2O \rightleftharpoons H_3O^+ + B^-$$

$$K_a = \frac{[H_3O^+][B^-]}{[HB]} \qquad .....(6.7)$$

In eq. 6.6 initial molar concentration of acetic acid is represented by 'c', concentration of $[H_3O^+]$ represented by x. The latter quantity equal to $[AC^-]$ because both ions formed in equimolar concentration. The concentration of acetic acid remaining at equilibrium [HAC] can be expressed as c-x. The reaction is

$$HAC + H_2O \rightleftharpoons H_3O^+ + AC^-$$
$$(c\text{-}x) \qquad\qquad x \quad\ x$$

and the equilibrium expression 6.6 becomes

$$K_a = \frac{x^2}{c - x} \qquad .....(6.8)$$

in this c is large in comparison $\bar{c}$ x. So the term c-x can be replaced by c.

$$K_a \cong \frac{x^2}{c}$$

which can be rearranged for calculation of hydrogen ion concentration of weak acids.

$$x^2 = K_a C$$

$$x = [H_3O^+] = \sqrt{K_a C}$$

$$x = \sqrt{K_a C} \qquad .....(6.9)$$

In general, for charged acids BH^+, the reaction is written

$$BH^+ + H_2O \rightleftharpoons H_3O^+ + B$$

The acidity constant is $K_a = \dfrac{[H_3O^+][B]}{[BH^+]}$

7. ***Ionization of weak bases***

Non-ionized weak bases B, exemplified by NH_3, react with water as

$$B + H_2O \rightleftharpoons OH^- + BH^+$$

$$K_b = \frac{[OH^-][BH^+]}{[B]} \qquad .....(6.10)$$

From the eq. 6.9 we can write $[OH^-] = \sqrt{K_bC}$ .....(6.11)

Salts of strong bases and weak acids, such as sodium acetate, dissociate completely in aqueous solution to give ions.

$$Na^+CH_3COO^- \xrightarrow{H_2O} Na^+ + CH_3COO^-$$

The sodium ions cannot react with H_2O as it would form NaOH, which is a strong electrolyte and would dissociate completely into ions. The acetate anion is weak base according to Bronsted-Lowry theory

$$CH_3COO^- + H_2O \rightleftharpoons OH^- + CH_3COOH$$

$$K_b = \frac{[OH^-][CH_3COOH]}{[CH_3COO^-]}$$

In general for an anionic base B^-,

$$B^- + H_2O \rightleftharpoons OH^- + HB$$

$$K_b = \frac{[OH^-][HB]}{[B^-]}$$ .....(6.12)

The acidity and basicity constants for a no. of pharmaceutically important acids and bases are listed in Tables 6.1 and 6.2. Last column gives dissociation exponent of P^K value, which is discussed later.

Table 6.1 Ionisation acidity constant for weak acids at 25 °C.

Weak acid	Molecular wt.	K_a	pK_a
Acetamino phen	151.16	1.20×10^{-10}	9.92
Acetic acid	60.05	1.75×10^{-5}	4.76
Acetyl salicylic acid	180.15	3.27×10^{-4}	3.49
Pamino benzoic	137.13	$K_1\ 2.24 \times 10^{-5}$	4.65
		$K_2\ 1.58 \times 10^{-5}$	4.80
Amino bacbital	226.27	1.15×10^{-8}	7.94
Ascorbic acid	176.12	$K_1\ 5 \times 10^{-5}$	4.3
		$K_2\ 1.6 \times 10^{-12}$	11.8
Benzoic acid	122.12	6.3×10^{-5}	4.20
Boric acid	61.84	5.8×10^{-10}	9.24
Benzyl pencillin	334.38	1.74×10^{-3}	2.76
Carbonic acid	44.01	$K_1\ 4.31 \times 10^{-7}$	6.37
		$K_2\ 4.7 \times 10^{-11}$	10.33

Citric acid (1 H$_2$O)	210.14	K$_1$ 7 × 10^{-4}	3.15
		K$_2$ 1.66 × 10^{-5}	4.78
		K$_3$ 4 × 10^{-7}	6.40
Formic acid	48.02	1.77 × 10^{-4}	3.75
Fumaric acid	116.07	K$_1$ 9.3 × 10^{-4}	3.03
		K$_2$ 4.2 × 10^{-5}	4.38
Gallic aicd	170.1	4 × 10^{-5}	4.4
α-D-Glucose	180.16	8.6 × 10^{-12}	12.1
Glycine	75.07	K$_1$ 4.5 × 10^{-3}	2.35
		K$_2$ 1.7 × 10^{-10}	9.78
Lactic acid	90.08	1.39 × 10^{-4}	3.86
Maleic acid	116.07	K$_1$ 1 × 10^{-2}	2.00
		K$_2$ 5.5 × 10^{-7}	6.26
Malic acid	134.09	K$_1$ 1 × 10^{-2}	3.4
		K$_3$ 9 × 10^{-6}	5.1
Malonic acid	104.06	K$_1$ 1.40 × 10^{-3}	2.85
		K$_2$ 2.0 × 10^{-6}	5.70
Mandelic acid	152.14	4.29 × 10^{-4}	3.37
Oxalic acid (2H$_2$O)	126.07	K$_1$ 5.5 × 10^{-2}	1.26
		K$_2$ 5.3 × 10^{-5}	4.28
Pencillin V	350.38	1.86 × 10^{-3}	2.73
Phenol	95.12	1 × 10^{-10}	10
Phospheric acid	98.00	K$_1$ 7.5 × 10^{-3}	2.12
		K$_2$ 6.2 × 10^{-8}	7.21
		K$_3$ 2.1 × 10^{-13}	12.67
Picric acid	229.11	4.2 × 10^{-1}	0.38
Salicylic acid	138.12	1.06 × 10^{-3}	2.97
Succinic acid	118.09	K$_1$ 6.4 × 10^{-5}	4.19
		K$_2$ 2.3 × 10^{-6}	5.63
Sucrose	342.30	2.4 × 10^{-13} (19 °C)	12.62
Sulfadiazine	250.28	3.3 × 10^{-7}	6.48
Sulfathiazole	255.32	7.6 × 10^{-8}	7.12
Tartaric acid	150.09	K$_1$ 9.6 × 10^{-4}	3.02
		K$_2$ 4.4 × 10^{-5}	4.36
Trichloro acetic acid	163.40	1.3 × 10^{-1}	0.89
Valeric acid	102.13	1.56 × 10^{-5}	4.81

Table 6.2 Ionization of basicity constants for weak bases at 25 $^{\circ}$C.

Weak base	Mol. wt	K_b	pK_b	pK_a (conjugated acid)
Acetanilide	135.16	4.1×10^{-14} (40 $^{\circ}$C)	13.39	0.61
Ammonia	35.05	1.74×10^{-5}	4.76	9.24
Atropine	289.4	4.5×10^{-5}	4.35	9.65
Benzo caine	165.19	6×10^{-12}	11.22	2.78
Caffaine	194.19	$K_1\ 3.98 \times 10^{-11}$	10.4	3.6
		$K_2\ 4.07 \times 10^{-14}$	13.4	0.6
Cocaine	303.35	2.6×10^{-6}	5.59	8.41
Codeine	299.36	1.6×10^{-6}	5.8	8.2
Ephedrine	165.23	2.3×10^{-5}	4.64	9.36
Epinephrine	183.20	$K_1\ 7.9 \times 10^{-5}$	4.1	9.9
		$K_2\ 3.2 \times 10^{-6}$	5.5	8.5
Erythromycin	733.92	6.3×10^{-6}	5.2	8.8
Ethylene diamine	60.10	7.1×10^{-8}	7.15	6.85
Glycine	75.07	2.3×10^{-12}	11.65	2.35
Morphine	285.33	7.4×10^{-7}	6.13	7.87
Procaine	236.30	7×10^{-6}	5.2	8.8
Pyridine	79.10	1.4×10^{-9}	8.85	5.15
Quinacrine (dihydrochloride)	472.88	1.0×10^{-6}	6.0	8.0
Strychinine	334.40	$K_1\ 1 \times 10^{-6}$	6.0	8.0
		$K_2\ 2 \times 10^{-12}$	11.7	2.3
Theobromine	180.17	$K_1\ 7.76 \times 10^{-7}$	6.11	7.89
		$K_2\ 4.8 \times 10^{-14}$	13.3	0.7
Theophylline	180.17	$K_1\ 1.58 \times 10^{-9}$	8.80	5.20
		$K_2\ 5.0 \times 10^{-14}$	13.3	0.7
Thiourea	76.12	1.25×10^{-12}	11.90	2.1
Urea	60.06	1.5×10^{-14}	13.82	0.18

6.2   Ionization of water

The concentration of hydrogen or hydroxyl ions in solutions or acids or bases may be expressed as gram ions/lt or as moles/lt.

A solution containing 17.008 gm of hydroxyl ions or 1.008 gm of hydrogen ions per lt. is said to contain 1 gm ion or 1 mole of hydroxyl or hydrogen ions per liter. A quantitative relationship between hydrogen is hydroxyl ions concentrations of any aqueous solution explains the ionization of water. The concentration of either the hydrogen or hydroxyl ions in acidic, neutral or basic solutions is usually expressed in terms of hydrogen ionic concentration or more conveniently in pH units.

Water ionizes slightly to yield hydrogen and hydroxyl ions. A weak electrolyte requires the presence of water or some other polar solvent for ionization. One molecule of water can be though of as a weak electrolytic solute that reacts with another molecule of water as the solvent. This auto protolytic reaction is expressed as

$$H_2O + H_2O \rightleftharpoons H_2O^+ + OH^-$$

The law of mass action is then applied to give the equilibrium expression

$$\frac{[H_3O^+][OH^-]}{[H_2O]^2} = K \qquad \qquad .....(6.13)$$

As molecular water exists in great excess relative to the concentration of hydrogen and hydroxyl ions $[H_2O]^2$ is considered as a constant and is combined with K to give a new constant, K_w known as dissociation constant, the autoprotolysis constant or the ion product of water.

$$K_w = K \times [H_2O]^2 \qquad \qquad .....(6.14)$$

The value of ion product is approximately 1×10^{-14} at 25 °C, it depends strongly on temperature.

Substituting the eq. 6.14 into 6.13 gives the common expression for the ionization of water.

$$[H_3O^+] \times [OH^-] K_w \cong 1 \times 10 - 14 \quad 25\,^{\circ}C \qquad \qquad .....(6.15)$$

In pure water, the hydrogen and hydroxyl ion concentration are equal and each has the value of approximately 1×10^{-7} mole/lt at 25 °C

$$[H_3O^+] \times [OH^-] \cong \sqrt{1 \times 10^{-14}}$$

$$\cong 1 \times 10^{-7} \qquad \qquad .....(6.16)$$

When an acid is added to pure water, some hydroxyl ions, provided by ionization of water, must always remain. The increase in hydrogen ions is compensated by a decrease in hydroxyl ions so k_w remains constant at about 1×10^{-14} at 25 °C.

1. *Relationship between K_a and K_b*

A relationship exists between dissociation constant of a weak acid HB and that of its conjugate base B^- or between BH^+ and B, when solvent is amphiprotic. This is obtained by multiplying eq. 6.7 by eq. 6.12.

$$K_a.K_b = \frac{\left[H_3O^+\right]\left[B^-\right]}{\left[HB\right]} \cdot \frac{\left[OH^-\right]\left[HB\right]}{\left[B^-\right]}$$

$$= \left[H_3O^+\right]\left[OH^-\right] = K_w$$

$$K_b = \frac{K_w}{K_a} \qquad\qquad .....(6.17)$$

$$K_a = \frac{K_w}{K_b} \qquad\qquad .....(6.18)$$

2. *Ionization of polyprotic electrolytes*

Acids that donate single proton and bases that accept a single proton are called monoprotic electrolytes. A polyprotic acid is one that is capable of donating 2 or more protons and a polyprotic base is capable of accepting 2 or more protons. Adiprotic acid, such as carbonic acid, ionizes in 2 stages and a triprotic (tribasic) acid such as phosphoric acid, ionizes in 3 stages. The equilibria involved in the protolysis or ionization of phosphoric acid together with the equilibrium expressions are

$$H_3PO_4 + H_2O = H_3O^+ + H_2PO_4^-$$

$$\frac{\left[H_3O^+\right]\left[H_2\,PO_4^-\right]}{\left[H_3\,PO_4\right]} = K_1 = 7.5\times10^{-3}$$

$$H_2PO_4^- + H_2O = H_3O^4 + HPO_4^{2-}$$

$$\frac{\left[H_3O^+\right]\left[HPO_4^{2-}\right]}{\left[H_2PO_4^-\right]} = K_2 = 6.2\times10^{-8}$$

$$HPO_4^{2-} + H_2O = H_3O^+ + PO_4^{3-}$$

$$\frac{\left[H_3O^+\right]\left[PO_4^{3-}\right]}{\left[H\,PO_4^{2-}\right]} = K_3 = 2.1\times10^{-13}$$

In any polyprotic electrolyte, the primary protolysis is greatest, and succeeding stages become less complete at any given acid concentration. Phosphoric acid is weak in the third stage of ionization and a solution of this acid contains practically no PO_4^{3-} ions.

Each of the species formed by the ionization of polyprotic acid can also act as a base. Thus for the phosphoric acid system

$$PO_4^{3-} + H_2O \rightleftharpoons HPO_4^{2-} + OH^-$$

$$K_{b1} = \frac{[HPO_4^{2-}][OH^-]}{[PO_4^{3-}]} = 4.8 \times 10^{-2}$$

$$HPO_4^{2} + H_2O \rightleftharpoons H_2PO_4^- + OH^-$$

$$K_{b2} = \frac{[H_2PO_4^-][OH^-]}{[HPO_4^{2-}]} = 1.6 \times 10^{-7}$$

$$H_2PO_4^- + H_2O \rightleftharpoons H_3PO_4 + OH^-$$

$$K_{b3} = \frac{[H_3PO_4][OH^-]}{[H_2PO_4^-]} = 1.3 \times 10^{-12}$$

For a polyprotic acid system for which the parent acid is H_nA there are n+1 possible species in solution.

$$H_{n-j}A + H_{n-j}A^{-i} + ... + HA^{-(n-1)} + A^{n-}$$

j represents no. of protons dissociated from parent acid and goes from 0 to n. The total concentration of all species must be equal to Ca, or

$$[H_nA] + [H_{n-j}A^{-j}] + ... + [H_A^{-(n-1)}] + [A^{n-}] = Ca$$

Each of the species pairs in which j differs by constitutes a conjugate acid-base pair and in general.

$$K_j \times K_{b(n+1-j)} = K_w$$

K_j represents various acidity constants, for phosphoric acid system described by equations.

$$K_1 K_{b3} = K_2 K_{b2} = K_3 K_{b1} = K_w$$

Ampholytes

In phosphoric acid system, the species $H_2PO_4^-$ and HPO_4^{2-} can function either as an acid or a base. A species that can function either as an acid or as a base is called an ampholyte and is to be amphoteric in nature. In general for a polyprotic acid system, all the species with the exception of $H_n A$ and A^{n-} are amphoteric. Amino acids and proteins are ampholytes. If glycine hydrochloride is dissolved in water, it ionizes as follows:

$$^+NH_3CH_2COOH + H_2O \rightleftharpoons \; ^+NH_3CH_2COO^- + H_3O^+$$

$$^+NH_3CH_2COO^- + H_2O \rightleftharpoons \; ^+NH_3CH_2COO + H_3O^+$$

The species $^+NH_3CH_2COO^-$ is amphoteric, these equations represents the reacting as an acid, it can react as a base with water as the follows:

$$^+NH_3CH_2COO^- + H_2O \rightleftharpoons \; ^+NH_3CH_2COOH + OH^-$$

The amphoteric species $^+NH_3CH_2COO^-$ is called a zwitter ion and differs from the amphoteric species formed from phosphoric acid in that it carries both a +ve and a −ve charge and the whole molecule is electrically neutral. The pH at which the zwittee ion concentration is a maximum is known as isoelectric point.

6.3 Sorenson's pH

The hydrogen ion concentration of a solution varies from approximately 1 in a 1 M solution of a strong acid to about 1×10^{-14} in a 1 M solution of a strong base. To compensate this difficulty, Sorensen suggested a simplified method of expressing Hydrogen ion concentration. He established the term pH which was originally written as p_H^+ to represent the hydrogen ion potential and he defined it as the common logarithm of the reciprocal of hydrogen ion concentration.

$$pH = \log \frac{1}{\left[H_3O^+\right]} \qquad \qquad .....(6.19)$$

$$pH = \log 1 - \log \left[H_3O^+\right]$$

as logarithm of 1 is zero, $pH = -\log \left[H_3O^+\right]$ $\qquad\qquad .....(6.20)$

The pH of a solution can be considered in terms of a numeric scale having values from 0 to 14 which expresses the acidity (7 to 0) and alkalinity (7 to 14). The value and at which the hydrogen and hydroxyl ion concentration are about equal at room temperature is referred to as neutral point or neutrality. The neutral pH at $^{\circ}$C is 7.47 and at 100 $^{\circ}$C it is 6.15.

Ion product of Water at Various Temperatures

Temperature ($^{\circ}$C)	$K_w \times 10^{14}$	pK_w
0	0.1139	14.944
10	0.2920	14.535
20	0.6809	14.167
24	1.000	14.000
25	1.000	13.007
30	1.469	13.833
37	2.57	13.59
40	2.919	13.535
50	5.474	13.262
60	9.614	13.017
70	15.1	12.82
80	23.4	12.63
90	35.5	12.45
100	51.3	12.29
300	400	11.40

The pH scale and corresponding Hydrogen and Hydroxyl ion concentrations.

pH	$[H_3O^+]$ (moles/lt)	$[OH^{-1}]$ (moles/lt)	
0	$10^0 = 1$	10^{-14}	↑
1	10^{-1}	10^{-13}	Acidic
2	10^{-2}	10^{-12}	↓
3	10^{-3}	10^{-11}	
4	10^{-4}	10^{-10}	↓
5	10^{-5}	10^{-9}	Neutral
6	10^{-6}	10^{-8}	↓
7	10^{-7}	10^{-7}	
8	10^{-8}	10^{-6}	
9	10^{-9}	10^{-5}	↑
10	10^{-10}	10^{-4}	
11	10^{-11}	10^{-3}	Basic
12	10^{-12}	10^{-2}	
13	10^{-13}	10^{-1}	↓
14	10^{-14}	$10^0 = 1$	

A better definition of pH involves the acidity activity rather than the concentration of the ions.

$$pH = - \log a\,H^+$$

Because the activity of an ion is equal to activity coefficient multiplied by the molal or molar concentration.

Hydronium ion concentration $\times$ Activity coefficient = Hydronium ion activity

pH may be computed more accurately from the formula.

$$pH = - \log (V \pm \times C)$$

The addition of a neutral salt affects the hydrogen ion activity of a solution and activity coefficients should be used for accurate calculations of pH.

1. ***Pharmaceutical significance of pH***

   Four principal types of pH, dependence of drug systems are – solubility, stability, activity and absorption.

   Drug solubility: If a salt, NaA is added to water to give a concentration C_s, the following reactions occur,

   $$Na^+ A^- \xrightarrow{\;H_2O\;} Na^+ + A^-$$

   $$A^- + H_2O \rightleftharpoons HA + OH^-$$

   In pH of the solution is lowered, more of the A^- would be converted to unionized acid, HA, from Lechatelice's principle. Sometimes a pH will be obtained below which the amount of HA formed exceeds its aqueous solubility and the acid will precipitate from solution. This pH can be designated as PHP. At this point at which the amount of HA formed just equals so, a mass balance on the total amount of drug is solution yields.

   $$C_s = [HA] + [A^-] = S_o + [A-]$$

   Replacing [A] as a function of hydronium ion concentration gives

   $$C_s = S_o + \frac{K_a C_s}{\left[H_3O^+\right]_p + K_a}$$

   K_a is ionization constant for conjugate acid HA, $[H_3O^+]_p$ is hydronium ion concentration above which precipitation will occur. This equation can be rearranged to give $\left[H_3O^+\right]_p = K_a \dfrac{S_o}{C_s - S_o}$

Upon taking logarithms it gives

$$-p_p^H = -\log K_a - \log \frac{C_s - S_o}{S_o}$$

$$p_p^H = pK_a + \log \frac{C_s - S_o}{S_o}$$

The analogous equation for salts of weak bases in strong acids (such as pilocarpine hydrochloride, cocaine hydrochloride and codeine phosphase) would be

$$p_p^H = pK_a + \log \frac{S_o}{C_s - S_o}$$

pK_a refers to protonated form of weak base.

Drug stability: The evidence for enhanced stability of systems when these are maintained within a narrow range of pH as well as of progressively decreasing stability as the pH departs from optimum range is abundant. Stability (or instability) of a system may result from gain or loss of a proton by a substrate molecule. Often acocompanied by an electronic rearrangement that reduces the reactivity of the molecule. Instability results when the substance desired to remain unchanged is converted to one or more other unwanted substances. In aqueous solution, instability may arise through a catalytic effect of acids or bases, the former by transferring a proton to the substrate molecule, the latter by accepting a proton. Morphine solutions are not decomposed. During a 60 min exposure at a temperature of 100 °C if pH is less than 5.5. Minimum hydrolytic decomposition of solutions of cocaine occurs in the range of pH 2.5. Thiamine hydrochloride is unstable above pH 5.

Drug activity: Often such drugs have as optimum pH range for maximum activity. Thus mandelic acid, Benzoic acid, salicylic acid have pronounced anti bacterial activity in non-ionized form but have practically no such activity in ionized form. These substances require an acid environment to function effectively as antibacterial agents. For ex. Sodium benzoate is effective as a preservative in 4% concentration at pH 7, in 0.06 to 0.1% concentration at pH 3.5 to 4 and in 0.02 to 0.03% concentration at pH 2.3 to 2.4. Acridines and quaternary ammonium compounds are active principally in cationic form.

Drug absorption: The degree of ionization and lipid solubility of drug are 2 important factors that determine the rate of absorption of drug. Drugs that are weak organic acids or bases and that in non ionized form are soluble in lipids, apparently are absorbed through cellular membrane by virtue of lipoidal nature of the membranes. pH determines the extent to which the drug will be converted to ionic or non ionic form become important parameters of drug absorption.

pH of purest water that is conductivity water is 7. Upon agitating this water in presence of CO_2 in atmosphere, the value drops rapidly to 5.7. This is the pH of nearly all distilled water, it is often called as "equilibrium" water.

Weakly acidic drugs exist primarily in un-ionised form in stomach (pH = 1 to 2). Their absorption will be excellent in acidic environment. Weakly basic drugs exist primarily in ionized form (conjugate acid) at the same site and their absorption will be poor. In the upper portion of small intestine, pH is more basic (5 to 7) and the reverse will be expected for weak acids and bases.

pH has considerable effect on stabilities and solubilities of many drugs, be injurious to body tissues and affect the case of absorption of drugs from gastrointestinal tract into the blood. Many drugs are weak bases or their salts. These drugs dissolve more rapidly in low pH of the acidic stomach. There will be little or no absorption of the drug as it will be too ionized. In alkaline intestine, ionization of dissolved base is reduced.

2. ***Conversion of pH to Hydrogen Ion Concentration***

Conversion of pH to hydrogen ion concentration can be illustrated as

$$pH = - \log [H_3O^+]$$

$$\log [H_3O^+] = - pH$$

$$[H_3O^+] = antilog\ (-pH)$$

p^H and p^{OH}: The use of pH to designate the negative logarithm of hydronium ion concentration has proved to be convenient that expressing numbers less than '1' in "p" notation has become a standard procedure. 'p' is a mathematical operator that acts on the quantity, $[H^+]$, K_a, K_b, K_w etc., to convert the value into the negative of its common logarithm. In other words, 'p' is used to express the negative logarithm of the term following the "p". For example p^{OH} express $-\log$ $[OH^-]$, p^{Ka} used to express $-\log$ Ka or p^{Kw} is $- \log$ Kw. From the equations and we can write,

$$p^H + p^{OH} = p^{Kw} \qquad \qquad .....(6.21)$$

$$pK_a + pK_b = p^{Kw} \qquad \qquad .....(6.22)$$

p^K is often called as the dissociation exponent. The p^K of weak acidic and basic drugs are ordinarily determined by ultra violet spectrophotometry and potentiometric titration. They may also be obtained by solubility analysis and by partition coefficient method. For ex. the reaction of a weakly acidic drug is

$$HA \rightleftharpoons H^+ + A^-$$

The ionization constant obtained by applying law of mass action is

$$K_a = \frac{[H^+][A^-]}{[HA]}$$

Taking logarithm on both sides

$$\log K_a = \log[H^+] + \log [A^-] - \log [HA]$$

By reversing the signs of this equation, we get

$$- \log K_a = -\log [H^+] - \log [A^-] + \log [HA]$$

As already we know, $- \log K_a = pK_a$, $- \log [H^+] = pH$. Substituting these in above equation, we get

$$pK_a = pH - \log [A^-] + \log [HA]$$

$$pK_a = pH + \log [HA] - \log [A^-]$$

$$pK_a = pH + \log \frac{[HA]}{[A^-]}$$

We can write a general equation for any acidic drug with one ionisable group, Cu is concentration of unionized species and Ci represents the concentration of ionized species. This is known as the "Henderson-Hasselbalch equation.

$$p^{Ka} = pH + \log \frac{Cu}{Ci} \qquad \qquad .....(6.23)$$

Similarly protonation of a weakly basic drug B can be represented by

$$B + H^+ \rightleftharpoons BH^+$$

The vase dissociation constant according to law of mass action is

$$K_b = \frac{[H^+][B]}{[BH^+]}$$

Upon taking negative logarithm, we get

$$p^{Kb} = pH$$

$$- \log K_a = - \log [A^+] - \log [B_-] + \log [BH^+]$$

$$p^{Kb} = pH + \log \frac{[BH^+]}{[B]}$$

The Henderson-Hasselbalch equation for any weak base with one ionisable group is written as,

$$p^{Kb} = pH + \log \frac{Ci}{Cu} \qquad \qquad .....(6.24)$$

where Ci and Cu refers to concentration of protonated and unionized species represented respectively. In potentiometric determination of ionization constants involves the titration of acid or base and application of Henderson equation.

$$pH = p^{Ka} + \log \frac{[Salt]}{[Acid]}$$

or $\qquad p^{Ka} = pH - \log \frac{[Salt]}{[Acid]}$

At 50 percent neutralisation i.e., when [salt] = [acid] then p^{Ka} = pH. This means that the ionization constant can be read directly from a titration curve simply by recording the pH at 50% neutralization.

6.4 The Influence of p^{Ka} Values on Transport of Drugs Across Biological Membranes

The ionized forms of acidic and basic drugs have low lipid: Water partition coefficients compared to coefficients for corresponding un-ionised molecules. So the lipid membranes are preferentially permeable to unionised molecules. Thus an increase in fraction of drug that is unionised will increase the rate of transport of drug across a lipid membrane. The Henderson-Hasselbalch equation indicates that the ratio of unionised : Ionised forms (Cu = Ci) of a given drug will depend on the pH of medium and the p^{Ka} value of the drug.

For example, the p^{Ka} value of aspirin which is a weak acid, is about 3.5 and if the pH of the gastric contents is 2.0 then

$$\log \frac{Cu}{Ci} = p^{Ka} - pH = 3.5 - 2.0 = 1.5$$

The ratio of concentration of unionised acetyl salicylic acid to acetyl salicylate anion is given by

$$Cu : Ci = \text{antilog } 1.5 = 31.62 : 1$$

Based on concentration of drug, for acidic drugs greater proportion of drug is absorbed into the plasma from stomach than from intestine. The reverse is true for basic drugs.

Species concentration as a function of pH

Polyprotic acids. HnA, can ionize in successive stages to yield n + 1 possible species in solution. In pharmaceutical studies, it is important to be able to calculate the concentration of all acidic and basic species in solution. The concentration of all species involved in successive acid-base equilibria change with pH and can be represented solely in terms of equilibrium constant and the hydronium ion concentration. These relationships can be obtained by defining all species in solution as fractions 'α' of total acid, Ca, added to system.

$$[H_nA] + [H_{n-i}A^{-p}] + \ldots + [HA^{-(n-1)}] + [A^{n-}] = Ca \text{ for poly protic acids}$$

$$\ldots..(6.25)$$

$$\alpha_0 = [H_nA]/Ca \qquad \ldots..(6.26)$$

$$\alpha_1 = [H_{n-1}A^{-1}]/Ca \qquad \ldots..(6.27)$$

In general
$$\alpha_j = [H_{n-j}A^{-p}]/Ca \qquad \ldots..(6.28)$$

and
$$\alpha_n = [A^{-n}]/Ca \qquad \ldots..(6.29)$$

j represents the no. of protons that have ionized from parent acid. Thus dividing eq. 6.25 by Ca and using equations 6.26 to 6.29 gives

$$\alpha_0 + \alpha_j + \ldots + \alpha_{n-1} + \alpha_0 = 1 \qquad \ldots..(6.30)$$

All of ∝ values can be defined in terms of equilibrium constant α_0 and $[H_3O^+]$ as follows

$$K_1 = \frac{[H_{n-1}A^-][H_3O^+]}{[H_nA]} = \frac{\alpha_1 \, Ca \, [H_3O^+]}{\alpha_0 \, Ca}$$

Therefore

$$\alpha_1 = \frac{K_1 \, \alpha_0}{[H_3O^+]} \qquad \ldots..(6.31)$$

$$K_2 = \frac{[H_{n-2}A^{2-}][H_3O^+]}{[H_{n-1}A^{1-}]} = \frac{[H_{n-2}A^{2-}][H_3O^+]^2}{K_1[H_nA]} = \frac{\alpha_2 \, Ca \, [H_3O^+]^2}{\alpha_0 \, Ca \, K_1}$$

$$\alpha_2 = \frac{K_1 \, K_2 \, \alpha_0}{[H_3O^+]^2} \qquad \ldots..(6.32)$$

In general
$$\alpha_j = \frac{(K_1 K_2 \ldots K_j)\alpha_o}{[H_3O^+]^j}$$
.....(6.33)

Inserting the appropriate forms of equation 6.33 into eq. 6.30 gives

$$\alpha_o + \frac{K_1 \alpha_o}{[H_3O^+]} + \frac{K_1 K_2 \alpha_o}{[H_3O^+]^2} + \ldots + \frac{K_1 K_2 \ldots K_n \alpha_o}{[H_3O^+]^n}$$

Solving for α_o yields

$$\alpha_o = \frac{[H_3O^+]^n}{\left\{[H_3O^+]^n + K_1[H_3O]^{n-1} + K_1 K_2 [H_3O^+]^{n-2} + \ldots + K_1 K_2 \ldots K_n\right\}}$$
.....(6.34)

or

$$\alpha_o = \frac{[H_3O^+]^n}{D}$$
.....(6.35)

D represents the denominator of eq. 6.34. Thus the concentration H_nA as a function of $[H_3O^+]$ can be obtained by substituting eq. 6.26 into eq. 6.35 to give

$$[H_nA] = \frac{[H_3O^+]^n Ca}{D}$$

Substituting eq. 6.27 into equation 6.35 gives and the resulting eq. into eq. 6.35 gives

$$[H_{n-1}A^{-1}] = \frac{K_1 [H_3O^+]^{n-1} Ca}{D}$$

In general
$$[H_{n-j}A^{-j}] = \frac{K_1 \ldots K_j [H_3O^+]^{n-j} Ca}{D}$$

and
$$[A^{-n}] = \frac{K_1 K_2 \ldots K_n Ca}{D}$$

For various types of poly protic acids

$$H_4A \Rightarrow D = [H_3O^+]^4 + K_1[H_3O^+]^3 + K_1 K_2[H_3O^+]^2 + K_1 K_2 K_3[H_3O^+] + K_1 K_2 K_3 K_4$$

$$H_3A \Rightarrow D = [H_3O^+]^3 + K_1[H_3O^+]^2 + K_1 K_2[H_3O^+] + K_1 K_2 K_3$$

$$H_2A \Rightarrow D = [H_3O^+]^2 + K_1[H_3O^+] + K_1 K_2$$

$$HA \Rightarrow D = [H_3O^+] + K_a$$

6.5 Calculation of pH

1. *Proton Balance equations*

In the Bronsted-Lowry system, the total number of protons released by a acidic species must equal to the total no. of protons consumed by basic species. This results in a very useful relationship known as the proton balance equation (PBE) in which the sum of the concentration terms for species that form by proton consumption is equated to sum of concentration terms for species that are formed by release of protons. The PBE forms the basis for pH calculations as it is an exact accounting of all proton transfer occurring in solution.

When HCl is added to water, for example, it dissociates yielding one Cl^- for each proton released. This Cl^- is a species formed by the release of a proton. In the same solution and actually in all aqueous solution.

$$2H_2O \rightleftharpoons H_3O^+ + OH^-$$

where H_3O^+ is formed by proton consumption and OH^- is formed by proton release. Thus the PBE is

$$[H_3O^+] = [OH^-] + [Cl^-]$$

General method for obtaining PBE is:

1. Start with species added to water

2. Place all species that can form when protons are released on the right side of the equation.

3. Place all species that can form when protons are consumed on the left side of the equation

4. Multiply the concentration of each species by no. of protons gained or lost to form that species.

5. Add $[H_3O^+]$ the left side of the equation and $[OH^-]$ to the right side of the equation. These result from interaction of 2 molecules of water as shown above.

What is the PBE when H_3PO_4 is added to water?

The species $H_2PO_4^-$ forms with the release of one proton.

The species HPO_4^{2-} forms with the release of 2 protons.

The species PO_4^{3-} forms with the release of 3 protons

We thus have

$$[H_3O^+] = [OH^-] + [H_2PO_4^-] + 2\left[HPO_4^{2-}\right] + 3\left[PO_4^{3-}\right]$$

What is the PBE when $Na_2 HPO_4$ is added to water?

The salt dissociates into $2 Na^+$ and one HPO_4^{2-}; Na^+ is neglected in the PBE because it is not formed from the release or consumption of a proton; HPO_4^{2-}, however, does react with water and is considered to be the starting species.

The species $H_2PO_4^-$ results with the consumption of one proton. The species of H_3PO_4 can form with the consumption of 2 protons.

The species PO_4^{3-} can form with the release of one proton.

Thus we have,

$$[H_3O^+] + [H_2 PO_4^-] + 2[H_3PO_4] = [OH^-] + \left[PO_4^{3-}\right]$$

2. *Solutions of strong acids and bases*

Strong acids and bases are those that have acidity or basicity constants greater than about 10^{-2}. Thus, they are considered to ionize 100% when placed in water. When HCl is placed in water, the PBE for the system is given by

$$[H_3O^+] = [OH^-] + [Cl^-] = \frac{K_w}{[H_3O^+]} + Ca$$

which can be arranged to give

$$\left[H_3O^+\right]^2 - Ca\left[H_3O^+\right] - K_w = 0 \qquad \qquad \text{.....(6.36)}$$

where Ca is the total acid concentration. This is a quadratic equation of the general form

$$ax^2 + bx + C = 0$$

which has the solution

$$x = \frac{-b \pm \sqrt{b^2 + 4ac}}{2a}$$

Thus eq. 6.36 becomes

$$\left[H_3O^+\right] = \frac{Ca + \sqrt{Ca^2 + 4K_w}}{2}$$

in which only the positive root is used because $[H_3O^+]$ can never be negative. When the concentration of acid is 1×10^{-6} M or greater $[Cl^-]$ becomes much greater than $[OH^-]$ in equation and Ca_2 becomes much greater than $4 K_w$ in equation. Thus, both equations simplify to

$$\left[H_3O^+\right] \cong Ca$$

A similar treatment for a solution of a strong base such as NaOH gives

$$[OH^-] = \frac{C_b + \sqrt{C_b^2 + 4\,K_w}}{2}$$

and
$$[OH^-] \cong C_b$$

If the concentration of base is 1×10^6 M or greater

3. Conjugate Acid-Base Pairs

PBE used to solve the pH of solutions composed of weak acids. Weak bases or a mixture of conjugate Acid-Base pair. Consider a solution made by dividing both a weak acid HB and a salt of its conjugate base, B⁻, in water. The acid-base equilibria involved are

$$HB + H_2O \rightleftharpoons H_3O^+ + B^-$$

$$B^- + H_2O \rightleftharpoons OH^- + HB$$

$$H_2O + H_2O \rightleftharpoons H_3O^+ + OH^-$$

PBE for this system is

$$[H_3O^+] + [HB] = [OH^-] + [B^-]$$

The concentration of acid and conjugate base may be expressed as

$$[HB] = \frac{[H_3O^+]\,C_b}{[H_3O^+] + K_a}$$

$$[B^-] = \frac{K_a\,Ca}{[H_3O^+] + K_a}$$

Table 6.1 Equivalent conductance of 25 $^{\circ}$C

S.No.	G.Eq/l	HCl	HOAC	NaCl	KCl	NaI	KI	NaoAC
1.	Inf. dil	426.1	390.6	126.5	149.9	126.9	150.3	91.0
2.	0.0005	422.7	67.7	124.5	147.8	125.4	–	89.2
3.	0.0010	421.4	49.2	123.7	146.9	124.3	-	88.5
4	0.0050	415.8	22.9	120.6	143.5	121.3	144.4	85.7
5.	0.0100	412.0	16.3	118.5	141.3	119.2	142.2	83.8
6.	0.0200	407.7	11.6	115.8	138.3	116.7	139.5	81.2
7.	0.0600	399.1	7.4	111.1	133.4	112.8	135.0	76.9
8.	0.1000	391.3	5.2	106.7	129.0	108.8	131.1	72.8

Table 6.2 Equivalent ion conductance at infinite dilution at 25 $^{\circ}$C.

S.No.	Cations	10	Anions	Co
1.	H^+	349.8	OH^-	198.0
2.	Li^+	38.7	Cl^-	76.6
3.	Na^+	50.1	Br^-	78.4
4.	K^+	73.5	I^-	76.8
5.	NH_4^+	61.9	ACO^-	40.9
6.	H_2Ca^{2+}	59.5	$\frac{1}{2}SO_4^{2}$	79.8
7.	$\frac{1}{2}\,Mg^{2+}$	53.0		

Table 6.3 Molality values of various compounds at various concentrations.

S.No.	Molality (m)	HCl	NaCl	NaOH	$Cacl_2$	H_2SO_4	Na_2SO_4	$CuSo_4$	$ZnSO_4$	KCl
1.	0.000	1.00	1.00	1.00	1.00	1.00	1.00	1.00	1.00	1.00
2.	0.005	0.93	0.93	-	0.73	0.64	0.78	0.53	0.48	0.93
3.	0.01	0.91	0.90	0.90	0.72	0.55	0.72	0.40	0.39	0.90
4.	0.05	0.83	0.82	0.81	0.58	0.34	0.51	0.21	0.20	0.82
5.	0.10	0.80	0.79	0.76	0.52	0.27	0.44	0.15	0.15	0.77
6.	0.50	0.77	0.68	0.68	0.51	0.16	0.21	0.067	0.063	0.65
7.	1.00	0.81	0.66	0.67	0.73	0.13	0.27	0.042	0.044	0.61
8.	2.00	1.01	0.67	0.69	1.55	0.13	0.15	-	0.035	0.58
9.	4.00	1.74	0.79	0.90	2.93	0.17	0.14	-	-	0.58

Table 6.4 Values of A and B for H_2O at various temperatures.

S.No.	Temperature (α)	A	B
1.	0	0.488	0.325×10^8
2.	15	0.500	0.328×10^8
3.	25	0.509	0.330×10^8
4.	40	0.524	0.333×10^8
5.	70	0.560	0.339×10^8
6.	100	0.606	0.348×10^8

Calculating Specific Conductance

1. When the electrolyte cell was filled with 0.01N Na_2SO_4 solution, it had a resistance of 397 ohm. What is the specific conductance? The electrolytic cell has a cell constant of 0.4460.

$$K = 0.4460$$

$$R = 397 \text{ ohm}$$

$$K = \frac{K}{R} = \frac{0.4460}{397} = 1.1234 \times 10^{3} \text{ mho/cm}$$

Specific and Equivalent Conductance

2. The measure conductance of 0.2 N solution of a drug is 0.0458 ohm at 25 $^{\circ}$C. The cell constant at 25 $^{\circ}$C is 0.630 cm^{-1}. What is the specific and equivalent conductance of the solution at this concentration?

$$C = 0.2 \text{ N} \qquad\qquad C = 0.0458$$

$$\text{Cell constant, } K = 0.630 \text{ cm}^{-1}$$

Specific conductance $\quad K = KC$

$$= 0.630 \times 0.0458$$

$$= 0.0288 \text{ mhol/cm}$$

Equivalent conductance, $\Lambda_c = K \times V$

$$= \frac{K \times 1000}{C} \text{ mho cm}^2/\text{eq}$$

$$= \frac{0.0288 \times 1000}{0.2}$$

$$= 144 \text{ mho cm}^2/\text{eq}$$

Osmotic Pressure of NaCl

3. What is the Osmotic pressure of 3.0 M solution of NaCl at 20 $^{\circ}$C? The I factor for NaCl is 1.9 (R = 0.082).

Van't Hoff $I = 19$

Gas constant $= R = 0.082$

Absolute temperature $T = 293$

Concentration, $C = 3.0 \text{ m}$

$$\pi = I \, RTC$$

$$= 1.9 \times 0.082 \times 293 \times 3.0$$

$$= 136.9 \text{ atm}$$

Degree of Dissociation

4. The equivalent conductance of acetic acid at 25 °C and at infinite dilution is 290.3 ohm/cm^2/eq. The equivalent conductance of a 5.9×10^3 N solution of acetic acid is 19.6 ohm cm^2/eq. What is the degree of dissociation of acetic acid at this concentration?

$$\Lambda_C = 19.6 \text{ ohm cm}^2/\text{eq}$$

$$\Lambda_o = 290.3 \text{ ohm cm}^2/\text{eq}$$

$$\propto = \frac{\Lambda_C}{\Lambda_o}$$

$$= \frac{19.6}{290.3} = 0.068 \text{ or } 6.8\%$$

Degree of Ionisation of Acetic acid

5. The freezing point of a 0.25 M solution of acetic acid is -0.743 °C. Calculate the degree of ionisation of acetic acid at the concentration. Acetic acid dissociate into two ions i.e., V = 2, (K_f = 61.86).

$$\Delta Tf = -0.743 \text{ °C}$$

$$Kf = 1.86$$

$$M = 0.25 \text{ m}$$

$$C = \frac{\Delta T_f}{K_f M} = \frac{0.743}{1.86 \times 0.25} = 1.599$$

$$\propto = \frac{i-1}{v-1}$$

$$= \frac{1.598-1}{2-1} = \frac{0.598}{1}$$

$$= 0.598$$

Mean Ionic Activity Co-efficient

6. Calculate the mean ionic activity co-efficient for 0.005 M atropine sulphate (1:2 electrolyte) in an aqueous solution containing 0.01 M Nacl at 25 °C. Because the drug is uni-bivalent electrolyte, $z_1 z_2 = 1 \times 2 = 2$. For water at 25 °C, A is 0.51.

$$\mu \text{ for atropine sulphate} = \frac{1}{2}[(0.005 \times 2 \times 1^2) + (0.005 \times 2^2)] = 0.015$$

$$\mu \text{ for Nacl} = \frac{1}{2}[(0.01 \times 1^2) + (0.01 + 1^2)] = 0.01$$

$$\mu = 0.015 + 0.01 = 0.025$$

$$\log r \pm = -0.51 \ Z_i^2 \ \sqrt{\mu} = -0.51 \times 2 \times \sqrt{0.025}$$

$$= -1.00 \times 0.158$$

$$\log r \pm = 0.158$$

$$r \pm = -(-0.802)$$

$$r \pm = 0.802$$

Osmolality

7. What is milliosmolality of 0.145 M solution of kBr? (i = 1.86)

$$\text{MIlliosmolality} = 1 \ mm$$

$$= 1.86 \times 0.145$$

$$= 26.97 \ mosm/kg$$

Osmolarity

8. A 0.154 M Nacl solution has a milliosmolarity of 29.67 mosm/kg. Calculate the milliosmolarity, M osm/l solution where density of the solvent water at 25 °C is $d_i^o = 0.9971$ g/cm and partial molal volume of solute –Nacl – is $\overline{V}_2^0 = 16.63$ ml/mole.

$$\text{Milliosmolarity} = (m \ osm/Kg \ H_2O) \times (d_i^o \ (1 - 0.001 \ \overline{V}_2^0))$$

$$= 2967 \times [0.9971 \ (1 - 0.001 \ (16.63))]$$

$$= 296.7 \times [0.9971 \ [1-0.01663]]$$

$$= 2967 \times [0.9971 \ (0.98337)]$$

$$= 296.7 \times [0.9805]$$

$$= 290.92 \ mosml/solution$$

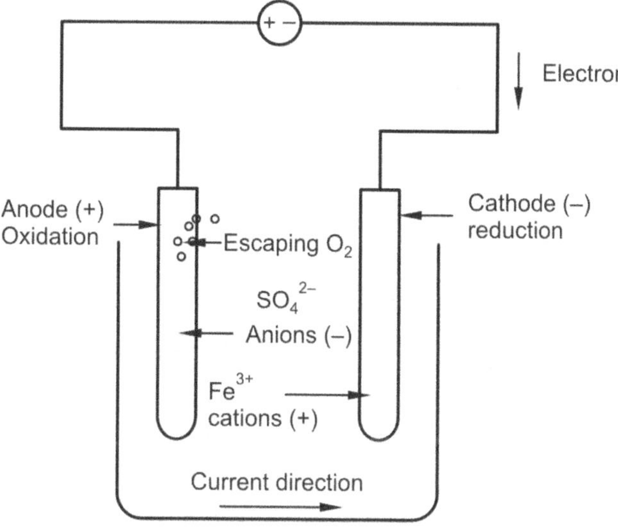

Fig. 6.1 Eletrolysis in electrolytic cell.

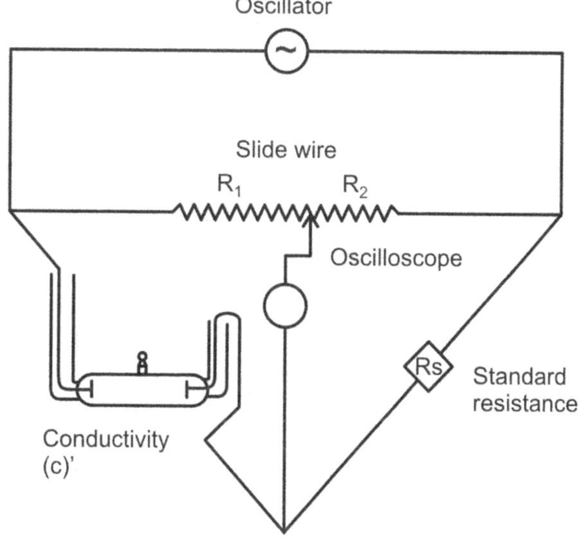

Fig. 6.2 Wheat stone bridge for measuring conductivity.

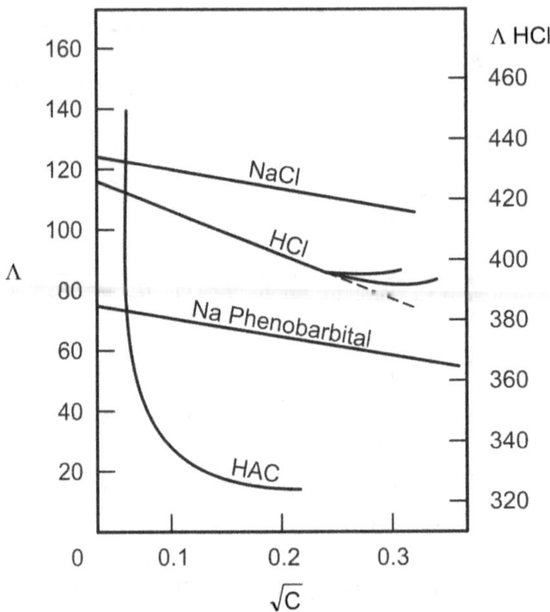

Fig. 6.3 Equivalent conductance of strong and weak electrolytes.

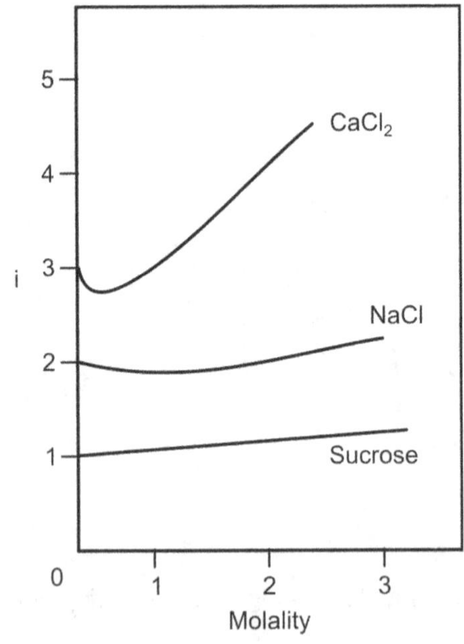

Fig. 6.4 Von't Hoff I factor of representative compound.

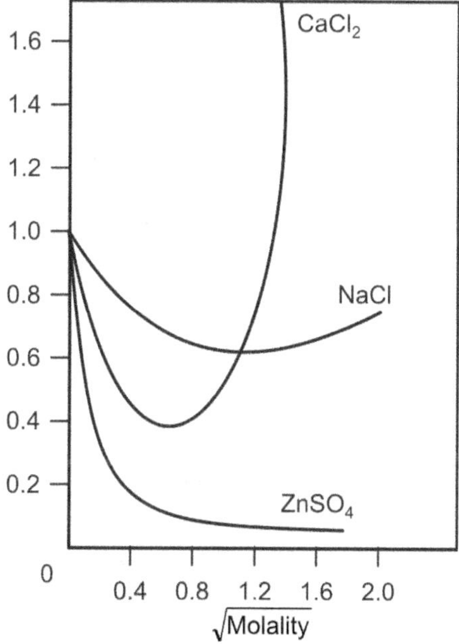

Fig. 6.5 Mean ionic activity co-efficient of representative electrolyte plotted against the square root of concentration.

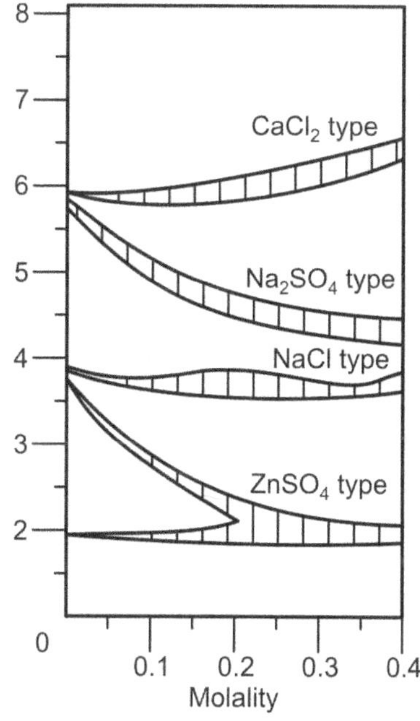

Fig. 6.6 L_{iso} values of ionic classes.

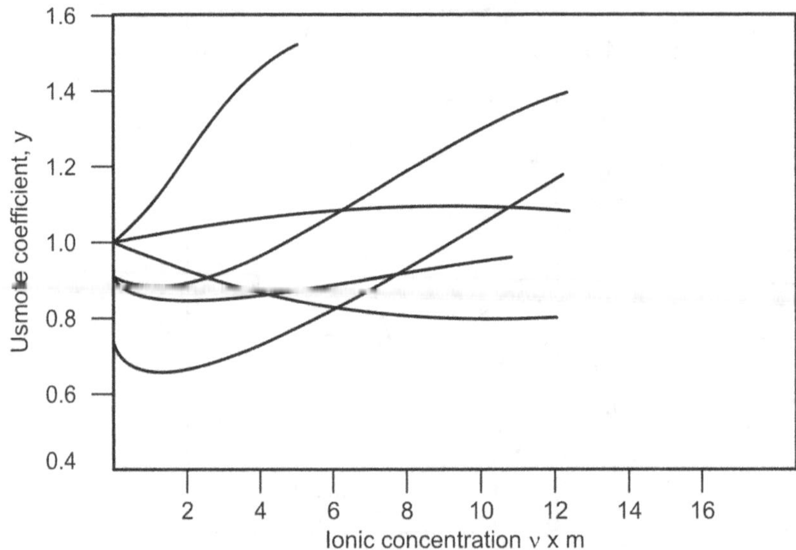

Fig. 6.7 Osmotic co-efficient for some common solutes.

6.6 Questions

1. Describe the theory of Acids and Bases.

2. What is pH and write about sorenson's pH scale and its importance in pharmacy.

CHAPTER 7

BUFFERS AND BUFFERED ISOTONIC SOLUTIONS

7.1 Introduction

7.1.1 Buffers

Buffers are compounds or mixture of compounds that, by their presence in solution, resist changes in pH upon addition of small quantities of acid or alkali. Hence they are used to maintain the pH level of a solution. The resistance to a change in pH is known as buffer action. If a small amount of strong acid or base is added to water or a solution of sodium chloride the pH is altered considerably, such systems have no buffer action. The pH value of buffer is slightly altered by addition of small amount of strong acid or base. The pH value of the buffer does not alter either on keeping for long periods or on dilution.

A combination of weak acid and its conjugate base (i.e., its salt) such as acetic acid and sodium acetate; or a weak base and its conjugate acid such as ammonium hydroxide and ammonium chloride, acts as a buffer. The buffers provide maximum stability of drugs against hydrolytic degradation or optimal solubility of drug in solution. The appropriate choice of a buffer depends on the pH range in which drug in question is most stable. Commonly used buffer systems are acetates, citrates, phosphates and glutamates. Although buffers ensure pH stability, the buffer system can affect other properties such as solubility and kinetics. They can act as general-acid or general-base catalysts and cause degradation of drug substance.

Table 7.1 lists buffers commonly used in liquid pharmaceutical products and their pH ranges. Table 7.2 lists common buffer-systems used in parenteral products.

Table 7.1 Buffers commonly used in liquid pharmaceutical products.

Buffer	pH	Usual concentration %
Acetic acid and a salt	3.5 – 5.7	1 – 2
Citric acid and a salt	2.5 – 6	1 – 3
Glutamic acid	8.2 – 10.2	1 – 2
Phosphoric acid salts	6 – 8.2	0.8 – 2

Table 7.2 Common buffers used in small-volume parenteral products.

pH	Buffers system	Concentration %
3.5 – 5.7	Acetic acid-acetate	1 – 2
2.5–6.0	Citric acid – citrate	1 – 5
6.0 – 8.2	Phosphoric acid-phosphate	0.8 – 2
8.2-10.2	Glutamic acid-glutamate	1 – 2

7.1.2 Buffer Equation

(i) ***Buffer Equation for a Weak Acid and Its Slat:*** Buffer equation is used to calculate the pH of a buffer solution and the change in pH of solution up on addition of an acid or base. This equation is developed by considering the effect of a salt on ionization of a weak acid when the salt and the acid have an ion in common.

For example, when sodium acetate is added to acetic acid, the dissociation constant for weak acid

$$K_a = \frac{[H_3O^+][AC^-]}{[HAC]} = 1.75 \times 10^{-5} \qquad \dots(7.1)$$

The equilibrium is disturbed because acetate ion supplied by the salt increases the $[AC^-]$ term in numerator. Hence to reestablish the constant K_a, the $[H_3O^+]$ term instantaneously decreases.

Consequently ionization of acetic acid, is represented by addition of common ion, AC^-

$$HAC + H_2O \rightleftharpoons H_3O^+ + AC^- \qquad \dots(7.2)$$

This is an example of common ion effect.

pH of final solution is obtained by rearranging eq. (7.1).

$$[H_3O^+] = K_a \frac{[HAC]}{[AC^-]} \qquad .....(7.3)$$

If the acid is weak and ionises only slightly, the expression [HAC] may be considered to represent the total concentration of acid, [acid]. In slightly ionised acidic solution, [AC⁻] can be considered as having come entirely from the salt; hence [AC⁻] term can be replaced by [salt]. Hence eq. 7.3 becomes

$$\left[H_3O^+\right] = K_a \frac{[Acid]}{[Salt]} \qquad .....(7.4)$$

By applying negative log to above equation

$$- \log [H_3O^+] = - \log K_a - \log [Acid] + \log [salt] \qquad .....(7.5)$$

$$\Rightarrow \qquad pH = pK_a + \log \frac{[Salt]}{[Acid]} \qquad .....(7.6)$$

Eq. 7.6 is called as Buffer equation or Henderson-Hassel balch equation for weak acid and its salt.

(ii) ***Buffer Equation for a Weak Base and Its Salt:*** The buffer equation for solutions of weak bases and its corresponding salts can be derived analogous to that of weak acid buffers.

$$[OH^-] = K_b \frac{[Base]}{[Salt]} \qquad .....(7.7)$$

But [OH⁻] = Kw [H_3O^+]; by substituting this

$$pH = pK_w - pK_b + \log \frac{[Base]}{[Salt]} \qquad .....(7.8)$$

Buffer solutions are not generally prepared from weak base and their salts because of volatility and instability of bases and because of dependence of their pH on pK_a which is often affected by temperature changes.

7.1.3 Buffer Equation and Activity Coefficients

Replacement of concentrations by activities in the equilibrium of a weak acid gives more exact equation for buffers

$$K_a = \frac{a_{H_3O^+}\, a_{AC^-}}{a_{HAC}} \qquad .....(7.9)$$

The activity of each species is written as the activity co-efficient multiplied by molar concentration

$$K_a = \frac{\left(\gamma_{H_3O^+}\, C_{H_3O^+}\right) \times \left(\gamma_{AC^-}\, C_{AC^-}\right)}{\gamma_{HAC}\, C_{HAC}} \qquad \text{.....(7.10)}$$

The activity coefficient of un-dissociated acid, γ_{HAC} is essentially

$$a_{H_3O^+} = \gamma_{H_3O^+} \times C_{H_3O^+} = K_a\, \frac{C_{HAC}}{\gamma_{AC^-}\, C_{AC-}} \qquad \text{.....(7.11)}$$

Applying – log to the above equation gives pH and hydrogen ion activity. pH defined as $- \log a_{H_3O^+}$

$$pH = pK_a + \log \frac{[Salt]}{[Acid]} + \log \gamma\, \overline{AC} \qquad \text{.....(7.12)}$$

From Debye-Huckel equation, for an aqueous solution of a univalent ion having ionic strength not greater than 0.1 or 0.2, at 25 °C

$$\text{Log } \gamma_{AC-} = \frac{-0.5\sqrt{\mu}}{1+\sqrt{\mu}}$$

Now eq. 7.12 becomes

$$pH = pK_a + \log \frac{[Salt]}{[Acid]} - \frac{0.5\sqrt{\mu}}{1+\sqrt{\mu}} \qquad \text{.....(7.13)}$$

General equation for buffers of polybasic acid is

$$pH = pK_n + \log \frac{[Salt]}{[Acid]} - \frac{A(2n-1)\sqrt{\mu}}{1+\sqrt{\mu}} \qquad \text{.....(7.14)}$$

where n is stage of ionization

7.1.4 Factors Influencing The pH of Buffer Solutions

The addition of neutral salts to buffers changes the pH of the solution by altering the ionic strength, hence pH changes. The addition of water in moderate amounts alters activity coefficients and may cause small positive or negative deviation. Bates expressed this quantitatively in terms of a dilution value. Dilution value is defined as change in pH on diluting the buffer solution to half of its original strength. A positive dilution value signifies that pH rises with dilution and vice-versa.

Temperature also influences buffers. Temperature coefficient of pH is the change in pH with temperature. The pH of acetate buffers was found to increase with temperature, whereas the pH of boric acid-sodium borate buffers decreases with temperature. The temperature coefficient of acid buffers was relatively small, that of basic buffers was large.

Drugs as Buffers

Solutions of drugs that are weak electrolytes posess buffer action. Salicylic acid solution when stored in a soft glass bottle, the sodium ions of the soft glass combine with salicylate ions to form sodium salicylate. The solution of salicyclic acid and sodium salicylate acts as a buffer solution. Similarly ephedrine and ephedrine hydrochloride also acts as buffer solution. Hence a drug in solution may often acts as its own buffer over a definite pH range.

pH Indicators

Indicators may be considered as weak acids or weak bases that act like buffers and exhibit colour changes as their degree of dissociation varies with pH. Buffers can be mixed to cover a wide pH range to yield universal indicators. The Merck Index suggests one universal indicator consisting of mixture of methyl yellow, methyl red, bromthymol blue, thymol blue and phenolphthalein that covers the range from pH 1 to 11. As indicators themselves are acids or bases, their addition to unbuffered solutions changes the pH of solution. However, some unbuffered solutions are buffered by the presence of drug itself and can withstand the addition of an indicator without significant change in pH.

Buffer Capacity

Buffer capacity is defined as the ratio of increment of strong base or acid to the small change in pH brought about by this addition

$$\beta = \frac{\Delta B}{\Delta pH} \qquad \qquad .....(7.15)$$

ΔB is small increment in gram equivalent/liter of strong base added to buffer solution. According to above equation, buffer capacity has a value of 1 when the addition of 1 gram eq. of strong base or acid to 1 liter of buffer solution results in change of 1 pH unit.

Buffers employed should have as low buffer capacity so as not to disturb the body's buffering systems, when injected into the body.

7.1.5 Calculation of Buffer Capacity

Consider an acetate buffer containing 0.1 mole each of acetic acid and sodium acetate in 1 liter of solution. To this 0.01 mole protons of sodium hydroxide are added. When the first increment of sodium hydroxide is added, the concentration of sodium acetate, the [salt] term in the buffer equation increases 0.01 mole/liter.

The acetic acid concentration, [Acid] decreases proportionately because each addition of base converts 0.01 mole of acetic acid into 0.01 mole of sodium acetate.

The reaction may be represented as

$$\underset{(0.1-0.01)}{HAC} + \underset{(0.01)}{NaOH} \rightleftharpoons \underset{(0.1+0.01)}{NaAc} + H_2O \qquad .....(7.16)$$

The changes in concentration of the salt and acid by the addition of a base are represented as

$$pH = pK_a + \log \frac{[Salt]+[Base]}{[Acid]-[Base]} \qquad .....(7.17)$$

The eq. 7.17 is used to verify the pH values and buffer capacities

Table 7.3 shows the results of pH of continual addition of sodium hydroxide.

Table 7.3 Buffer capacity of solutions containing equi-molar amounts of (0.1 M) Acetic acid and sodium acetate.

Moles of NaOH added	pH of solution	Buffer capacity, β
0	4.76	
0.01	4.85	0.11
0.02	4.94	0.11
0.03	5.03	0.11
0.04	5.13	0.10
0.05	5.24	0.09
0.06	5.36	0.08

Buffer capacity is not a fixed value for a given buffer system, but depends on the amount of base added. Buffer capacity changes as the ratio log ([Salt]/ [Acid]) increases with addition of base, the buffer capacity deceases rapidly. Buffer has greatest capacity when [salt]/ [Acid] = 1 i.e., when pH = pK_a. Concentration also influences buffers capacity. In a weak acid/conjugate base buffer, the concentration of salt determines capacity to neutralize the added acid. Greater the concentration of salt and acid, greater the alkaline and acid reserve.

Exact Equation for Buffer Capacity

Vanslyke and Koppel and Spiro developed a more exact equation

$$\beta = 2.3\,C\frac{K_a\left[H_3O^+\right]}{\left(K_a + \left[H_3O^+\right]\right)^2} \qquad \qquad .....(7.18)$$

C is total buffer concentrations i.e., sum of molar concentrations of the acid and salt. This equation permits to compute the buffer capacity at any hydrogen ion concentration, at any point where no acid or bases has been added to the buffer.

Influence of Concentration on Buffer Capacity

Buffer capacity is affected not only by [Salt]/ [Acid] ratio, but also by concentrations of acid and salt. As shown in Table 7.3 when 0.01 mole of base is added to a 0.1 molar acetate buffer, the pH increases from 4.76 to 4.85, ΔpH is 0.09.

If concentration of Acetate buffer is 1M, the pH of original buffer solution remains at about 4.76, but up on addition of 0.01 mole of base, it becomes 4.77, ΔpH = 0.01

$$pH = 4.76 + \log\frac{1.0 + 0.01}{1.0 - 0.01} \qquad \qquad .....(7.19)$$

Therefore increase in concentration of buffer components results in greater buffer capacity.

Maximum Buffer Capacity

The maximum buffer capacity occurs where pH = pK_a where $[H_3O^+]$ = K_a. Substituting in eq. 7.18

$$\beta_{max} = 2.303\,C\frac{\left[H_3O^+\right]^2}{\left(2\left[H_3O^+\right]\right)^2} = \frac{2.303}{4}C$$

$$\beta_{max} = 0.576\,C \qquad \qquad .....(7.20)$$

where C = total buffer concentration

7.2 Neutralisation Curves and Buffer Capacity

Buffer capacity can be obtained by considering the titration curves of strong and weak acids when they are mixed with increasing quantities of alkali.

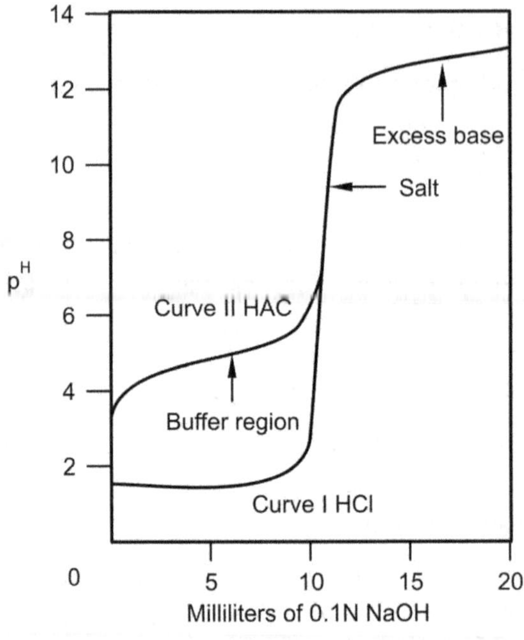

Fig. 7.1

The neutralization of 10 ml of 0.1N HCl and 10 ml of 0.1 N acetic acid by 0.1N NaOH is shown in Fig. 7.1. The plot of pH versus millimetres of NaOH added produces the titration curve. Before addition of NaOH the hydrogen ion concentration of 0.1 N HCl is 10^{-1} mole/liter and pH is 1. The addition of 5 ml of 0.1 N NaOH neutralizes 5 ml 0.1 N HCl, leaving 5 ml of original HCl in total 15 ml of solution. $[H_3O^+] = 5/15 \times 0.1 = 3.3 \times 10^{-2}$ mole/liter and pH is 1.48. When 10 ml of base is added, all HCl is converted to NaCl and pH is 7. This is known as equivalence point of titration.

It is seen that the pH does not change until all HCl is neutralized. Hence a solution of strong acid has high buffer capacity below pH 2.

Similarly a strong base has high buffer capacity above pH of 12.

The buffer capacity of solution of strong acid was directly proportional to hydrogen ion concentration, by Vanslyke equation

$$\beta = 2.303 \, [H_3O^+] \qquad\qquad\qquad \text{.....(7.21)}$$

The buffer capacity of solution of strong base is proportional to hydroxyl ion concentration

$$\beta = 2.303 \, [OH^-] \qquad\qquad\qquad \text{.....(7.22)}$$

The total buffer capacity of a solution of strong acid or base at any pH is sum of eq. 7.21 and 7.22

$$\beta = 2.303\ ([H_3O^+] + [OH^-]) \qquad \qquad .....(7.23)$$

Consider the addition of 0.1N NaOH to 10 ml of 0.1N HAC solution

(a) the pH of solution before NaOH has been added is obtained from equation for a weak acid

$$[H_3O^+] = \sqrt{K_a\ C_a}$$

$$pH = \frac{1}{2}pK_a - \frac{1}{2}\log C \qquad \qquad .....(7.24)$$

$$= 2.38 - \frac{1}{2}\log 10^{-1} = 2.88$$

(b) At equivalence point, the pH is obtained from the equation for a salt of weak acid and strong base

$$\left[H_3O^+\right] = \sqrt{\frac{K_a K_w}{C_b}}$$

$$pH = \frac{1}{2}\ pK_w + \frac{1}{2}PK_a + \frac{1}{2}\log C \qquad \qquad .....(7.25)$$

$$= 7.00 + 2.38 + \frac{1}{2}\log (5 \times 10^{-2})$$

$$= 8.73$$

Here the concentration of acid in this equation is 0.05 because the solution has been reduced to half of its original value by addition of equal volume of base at equivalence point.

(c) Between these points on Neutralization curve, the increments of NaOH convert some acid to its conjugate base to form a buffer mixture and pH of system is calculated from buffer equation. When 5 ml base is added, the equivalent of 5 ml of 0.1N acid remains and 5 ml of 0.1N AC$^-$ is formed

$$pH = pKa + \log \frac{[Salt]}{[Acid]}$$

$$= 4.76 + \log \frac{5}{5} = 4.76$$

The slope of curve is minimum and buffer capacity is greatest at this point; i.e., at half-neutralisation where $pH = pK_a$.

7.2.1 Buffers in Pharmaceutical and Biological System

In-Vivo Biological Buffer Systems

Blood is maintained at pH of 7.4 by primary buffers in plasma. Plasma contains carbonic acid/bicarbonate and acid/alkali sodium salts of phosphoric acid as buffers. The buffer capacity of blood is in physiological range of 7.0 to 7.8.

Zacrimal fluid, or tears have great degree of buffer capacity allowing dilution of 1:15. The pH of tears is about 7.4 with range of 7 to 8.

Urine has pH of about 6, with a range of 4.5 to 7.8.

Pharmaceutical Buffers

The Clark-Lubs mixtures used as buffers are

(a) HCl and KCl – pH 1.2 to 2.2

(b) HCl and potassium hydrogen phthalate – pH 2.2 to 4.0

(c) NaOH and potassium hydrogen phthalate – pH 4.2 to 5.2

(d) NaOH and KH_2PO_4 – pH 5.8 to 8.0

(e) H_3BO_3, NaOH and KCl – pH 8.0 to 10.0

Buffered Isotonic Solutions

In addition to carrying out pH adjustment, pharmaceutical solutions that are meant for application to delicate membranes of body should be adjusted to the same osmotic pressure as that of body fluids. Hence buffered isotonic solutions are used.

Measurement of Tonicity

There are 2 methods of measuring tonicity. First method is haemolytic method, the effect of various drug solutions on appearance of red blood cells suspended in solutions is observed. The second method is to measure Tonicity by using any of methods used to measure colligative properties. 0.09% NaCl solution is considered to be isotonic with both blood and lacrimal fluid.

7.2.2 Calculating Tonicity using L_{iso} Value

Because the freezing point depressions for solutions of electrolytes of both weak and strong types are always greater than those calculated from equation

$\Delta T_f = K_f C$, a new factor $L = iK_f$ is introduced in equation

$$\Delta T_f = LC \qquad\qquad .....(7.26)$$

The L value at a concentration C that is isotonic with body fluids is called L_{iso}.

The L_{iso} value for 0.9% solution of sodium chloride which has freezing point depression of 0.52 °C and isotonic with body fluids is 3.4 from

$$L_{iso} = \frac{\Delta T_f}{C} \qquad\qquad .....(7.27)$$

$$L_{iso} = \frac{0.52\ ^\circ C}{0.154} = 3.4$$

For dilute solutions of non-electrolytes L_{iso} is approximately equal to K_f. Table 7.3 is used to obtain ΔT_f for a solution of a drug. A plot of iK_f against molar concentration of various types of electrolytes is shown in Fig. 7.2.

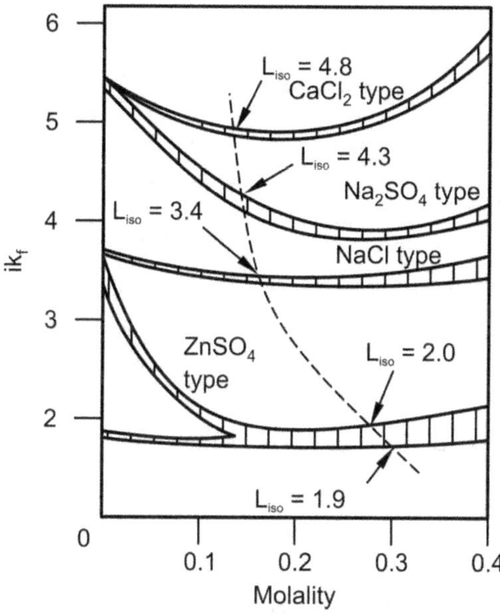

Fig. 7.2 Plot of iK_f against molar concentration of different types of electrolytes

7.3 Methods of Adjusting Tonicity and pH

To calculate the quantity of sodium chloride, dextrose and other substances that may be added to solutions of drugs to render them isotonic, there are 2 methods. Class I and Class II.

In class I methods, the sodium chloride or some other substance is added to drug solution to lower the freezing point of solution to -052 °C and thus make it isotonic with body fluids. There are 2 methods, cryoscopic method and sodium chloride equivalent method under class I. In class II methods, water is added to drug in sufficient amount to form an isotonic solution. Included methods in this class are white-vincent method and sprowls method. In these methods, the preparation is brought to its final volume with an isotonic or buffered isotonic dilution solution.

7.3.1 Class I Methods

7.3.1.1 *Cryoscopic Method:* The freezing point depressions of a number of drug solutions is determined experimentally or theoretically and given in Table 7.4. The drug solutions whose freezing point depressions are not previously determined can be calculated by knowing only molecular weight of drug and L_{iso} value of the ionic class.

Table 7.4 Freezing point depressions of drug solution

Drug substance	ΔTf	L_{iso}
Aminophylline	0.10	4.6
Atropine sulphate	0.11	1.9
Boric acid	0.29	1.8
Chloram phenicol	0.06	1.9
Calcium gluconate	0.09	4.2
Emetine hydrochloride	0.06	3.3
Ephedrine sulphate	0.14	5.8

7.3.2 Sodium Chloride Equivalent Method

This method was developed by Mellen and Seltzer. The 'Sodium Chloride Equivalent' or the 'Tonicic Equivalent' of a drug is the amount of sodium chloride that has same osmotic effect as that of 1 g, or other weight unit of the drug. The sodium chloride equivalents E for a number of drugs are listed in Table. The E value of a new drug can be calculated from L_{iso} value or freezing point depression of the drug. For a solution containing 1 g of drug in 1000 ml of solution, the concentration C in moles/liter can be calculated as

$$C = \frac{1\,g}{\text{Moleclar weight}} \qquad\qquad .....(7.28)$$

From equation

$$\Delta T_f = L_{iso}\,\frac{1\,g}{M\,W}$$

E is the weight of NaCl with same freezing point depression as 1g of drug,

$$\Delta T_f = 3.4\,\frac{E}{58.45} \qquad\qquad .....(7.29)$$

where 3.4 is L_{iso} value for sodium chloride and 58.45 is its molecular weight

$$\frac{L_{iso}}{MW} = 3.4 \frac{E}{58.45} \qquad \ldots(7.30)$$

$$E \cong 17 \frac{L_{iso}}{MW} \qquad \ldots(7.31)$$

The amount of sodium chloride or other inert substance required to make the solution isotonic is obtained as below.

White and Vincent developed this method and the explanation is as follows:

Suppose one needs to make 30 ml of a 1% solution of procaine hydrochloride isotonic with body fluid, the weight of the drug, W, is multiplied by sodium chloride equivalent, E

$$0.3 \times 0.21 = 0.063 \text{ g}$$

This is the quantity of sodium chloride osmotically equivalent to 0.3 g of procaine hydrochloride.

It is known that 0.9 g of sodium chloride when dissolved in enough water to make 100 ml yields a solution that is isotonic. The volume V, of isotonic solution that can be prepared from 0.063 g of sodium chloride is obtained by solving the proportion

$$\frac{0.9\,\text{g}}{100\,\text{ml}} = \frac{0.063\,\text{g}}{V} \qquad \ldots(7.32)$$

The quantity of drug in prescription is multiplied by its sodium chloride equivalent and this value is subtracted from concentration of sodium chloride that is isotonic with body fluids i.e., 0.9 g/100 ml. Other agents such as dextrose can be used to replace NaCl. The concentration of these agents for isotonicity is calculated by use of equation

$$X = \frac{Y\,(\text{additional amount of NaCl for isotonicity})}{E\,(\text{Grams of NaCl equivalent to 1 g of isotonic agent})}$$

where X is grams of isotonic agent required to adjust the tonicity.

7.3.3 Class II Methods

7.3.3.1 *White-Vincent method:* The class-II methods of adjusting tonicity involve the addition of water to drugs followed by addition of an isotonic or isotonic-buffered diluting vehicle to bring solution to final volume

$$V = 0.063 \times \frac{100}{0.9} \qquad \ldots(7.33)$$

$$V = 7.0 \text{ ml}$$

In eq. 7.33, the quantity 0.063 is equal to weight of drug W, multiplied by sodium chloride equivalent, E. The value of ratio 100/0.9 is 111.1. Now eq. 7.33 can be written as

$$V = W \times E \times 111.1 \qquad \ldots(7.34)$$

where V is volume in millilitres of isotonic solution, W is weight in grams of drug and E is sodium chloride equivalent. The constant, 111.1 represents volume in millilitres of isotonic solution obtained by dissolving 1 g of sodium chloride in water.

$$V = 0.3 \times 0.21 \times 111.1$$

$$= 7.0 \text{ ml}$$

To complete the isotonic solution enough isotonic sodium chloride solution, another isotonic solution or an isotonic buffered solution is added to make 30 ml of finished product. Several isotonic and isotonic-buffered diluting solutions are listed in Table 7.5. They have isotonicity values of 0.9% NaCl.

Table 7.5 Isotonic and Isotonic buffered solutions.

Isotonic diluting solutions	
Isotonic sodium chloride solution	USP
Dextrose solution	5.6%
Sodium nitrate solution	1.3%
Ringer's solution	USP
Diluting solution 1, pH 4.7	
Boric acid	20
Diluting solution II, pH 6.8	4.6 G
Sodium acid phosphate	
Diluting solution III, pH 7.4	
Disodium phosphate Anhydrous	8.1 G
Diluting solution IV, pH 9	
Sodium borate	4.2 G

Problems

pH Calculation

1. What is the pH of 0.1M acetic acid solution $pK_a = 4.76$? What is the pH after enough sodium acetate has been added to make the solution 0.1M with respect to its salt?

Sol: The pH of acetic acid is calculated by use of the logarithmic equation

$$[H_3O^+] = \sqrt{K_a C_a}$$

$$pH = \frac{1}{2}pK_a - \frac{1}{2}\log C$$

$$pH = 2.38 + 0.50 = 2.88$$

The pH of the buffer solution containing acetic acid and sodium acetate is determined by use of buffer equation

$$pH = pK_a + \log \frac{[Salt]}{[Acid]}$$

$$= 4.76 + \log \frac{0.1}{0.1} = 4.76$$

2. What is the pH of solution containing 0.10 mole of ephedrine and 0.01 mole of ephedrine hydrochloride per litre of solution? pK_b of Ephedrine is 4.64.

$$pH = pK_w - pK_b + \log \frac{[Base]}{[Salt]}$$

$$pH = 14 - 4.64 + \log \frac{0.10}{0.01}$$

$$pH = 9.36 + \log 10 = 10.36$$

Buffer Capacity

3. At a hydrogen ion concentration of 1.75×10^{-5} (pH = 4.76) what is the capacity of a buffer containing 0.10 mole each of acetic acid and sodium acetate per liter of solution? The total concentration of C= [Acid] + [Salt] is 0.20 mole/liter and dissociation constant is 1.75×10^{-5}.

$$\beta = \frac{2.3 \times 0.20 \times \left(1.75 \times 10^{-5}\right) \times \left(1.75 \times 10^{-5}\right)}{\left[\left(1.75 \times 10^{-5}\right) + \left(1.75 \times 10^{-5}\right)\right]^2}$$

$$= 0.115$$

4. What is the change of pH on adding 0.01 mole of NaOH to 1 L of 0.10 M acetic acid?

(a) Calculate the pH of a 0.10 molar solution of acetic acid

$$\left[H_3O^+\right] = \sqrt{K_a C_a} = \sqrt{1.75 \times 10^{-4} \times 1.0 \times 10^{-1}}$$

$$= 4.18 \times 10^{-3}$$

$$pH = -\log 4.18 \times 10^{-3} = 2.38$$

(b) on adding 0.01 mole of NaOH to a liter of this solution, 0.01 mole of acetic acid is converted to 0.01 mole of sodium acetate thereby decreasing C_a to 0.09 M and $C_b = 1.0 \times 10^{-2}$ M. Using Henderson-Hasselbalch equation gives

$$pH = 4.76 + \log \frac{0.01}{0.09}$$

$$= 4.76 - 0.95$$

$$= 3.81$$

The pH change is therefore, 1.43 units. The buffer capacity as defined above is calculated as

$$\frac{\text{Moles of NaOH added}}{\text{Change in pH}} = 0.011$$

Maximum Buffer Capacity

5. What is the maximum buffer capacity of an acetate buffer with a total concentration of 0.20 mole/liter?

$$\beta_{max} = 0.576 \ C$$

$$= 0.576 \times 0.02$$

$$= 0.01152$$

6. What is the buffer capacity of a solution of hydrochloric acid having a hydrogen ion concentration of 10^{-2} mole/liter.

   The hydroxyl ion concentration of such a solution is 10^{-12} and total buffer capacity is

$$\beta = 2.303 \ (10^{-2} + 10^{-12})$$

$$\beta = 0.023$$

Sodium Chloride Equivalents

7. Calculate the approximate E value for a new amphetamine hydrochloride derivative (molecular weight 187)

   Because this drug is univalent salt, L_{iso} value is 3.4. E value is calculated as

$$E = 17 \ \frac{L_{iso}}{MW}$$

$$= 17 \ \frac{3.4}{187} = 0.31$$

Tonicity Adjustment

8. A solution contains 1.0 g of ephedrine sulphate in a volume of 100 ml. What quantity of sodium chloride must be added to make the solution isotonic?

   The weight of sodium chloride to which the quantity of drug is equivalent is obtained by multiplying the quantity of drug by its sodium chloride equivalent E.

Ephedrine sulphate: $1.09 \times 0.23 = 0.23$ g

Ephedrine sulphate has contributed a weight of material osmotically equivalent to 0.23 g of sodium chloride. Because a total of 0.9 g of sodium chloride is required for isotonicity is

$$0.90 - 0.23 = 0.67 \text{ g}$$

7.4 Isotonic Solution

9. Make following solution isotonic with respect to an ideal membrane

Phenocaine hydrochloride   -   0.06 g

Boric acid   -   0.30 g

Sterilized distilled water enough to make 100.0 ml

$$V = [(0.06 \times 0.20) + (0.3 \times 0.50)] \times 111.1$$

$$V = 18 \text{ ml}$$

The drugs are mixed with water to make 18 ml of an isotonic solution, and the preparation is brought to a volume of 100 ml by adding an isotonic diluting solutions.

The equation $[HB] = \dfrac{[H_3O^+]C_b}{[H_3O^+]+K_a}$ contains C_b concentration of base added as the salt] rather than C_a because in terms of PBE, the species HB was generated from the species B^- added in the form of the salt equation $[B^-] = \dfrac{K_a C_a}{[H_3O^+]+K_a}$ contains C_a (concentration of HB added) because the species B^- in the PBE came from the HB added. Inserting these 2 equations into $[H_3O^+] + [HB] = [OH^-] + [B^-]$ gives

$$[H_3O^+] + \frac{[H_3O^+]C_b}{[H_3O^+]+K_a} = [OH^-] + \frac{K_a C_a}{[H_3O^+]+K_a}$$

up on rearrangement

$$[H_3O^+] = K_a \frac{\left(C_a - [H_3O^+] + [OH^-]\right)}{\left(C_b + [H_3O^+] - [OH^-]\right)} \qquad .....(7.35)$$

7.4.1 Solutions Containing Only a Weak Acid

If the solution contains only a weak acid, C_b is zero and $[H_3O^+]$ is generally much greater than $[OH^-]$. Thus eq. 7.35 is simplified to

$$[H_3O^+]^2 + K_a[H_3O^+] - K_a C_a = 0$$

This is a quadratic equation with solution

$$\left[H_3O^+\right] = \frac{-K_a + \sqrt{K_a^2 + 4K_aC_a}}{2} \qquad \dots(7.36)$$

In many instances, C_a is much greater than $[H_3O^+]$, so the equation can be simplified to

$$\left[H_3O^+\right] = \sqrt{K_aC_a} \qquad \dots(7.37)$$

The eq. 7.37 gives an answer for $[H_3O^+]$ with a relative error of 18% as compared with the correct answer given by the eq. 7.36.

7.4.2 Solutions Containing Only a Weak Base

If the solution contains only a weak base, C_a is zero and $[OH^-]$ is generally much greater than $[H_3O^+]$. Thus the eq. 7.35 can be simplified to

$$\left[H_3O^+\right] = \frac{K_a\left[OH^-\right]}{C_b - \left[OH^-\right]} = \frac{K_a K_w}{\left[H_3O^+\right]C_b - K_w} \qquad \dots(7.38)$$

This equation can be solved for either $[H_3O^+]$ or $[OH^-]$. If we solve for $[H_3O^+]$, it gives
$$C_b\,[H_3O^+]^2 - K_w\,[H_3O^+] - K_a K_w = 0$$

which has the solution

$$\left[H_3O^+\right] = \frac{K_w + \sqrt{K_w^2 + 4C_b K_a K_w}}{2\,C_b}$$

If K_a is much greater than $[H_3O^+]$ which is true for solutions of weak bases, we get an equation

$$\left[H_3O^+\right] = \sqrt{\frac{K_a K_w}{C_b}}$$

If the eq. 7.38 is solved for $[OH^-]$, by converting K_a to K_b to give

$$\left[OH^-\right] = \frac{-K_b + \sqrt{K_b^2 + 4 K_b C_b}}{2}$$

and if C_b is much greater than $[OH^-]$, which generally true for solutions of weak bases, we get

$$\left[OH^-\right] = \sqrt{K_b\,C_b}$$

7.4.3 Solutions Containing a Single Conjugate Acid-Base Pair

If a solution composed of a weak acid and a salt of that acid (e.g., acetic acid and sodium acetate) or a weak base and a salt of that base (e.g., ephedrine and ephedrine hydrochloride). C_a and C_b are generally much greater than either $[H_3O^+]$ or $[OH^-]$, thus the eq. 7.35 can be simplified to

$$\left[H_3O^+\right] = \frac{K_a\,C_a}{C_b}$$

The solutions made by dissolving in water, both an acid and its conjugate base or a base and its conjugate acid are the examples of buffer solutions. These solutions are of great importance in pharmacy.

7.4.4 Two Conjugate Acid-Base Pairs

The Bronsted-Lowry theory and the PBE, enable a single equation to be developed that is valid for solutions containing an ampholyte which forms a part of 2 dependent acid-base pairs. An amphoteric spheres can be added directly to water or it can be formed by the reaction of a diprotic weak acid H_2A or a diprotic weak base, A^{2-} substances such as $NaHCO_3$ and NaH_2PO_4 are termed as ampholytes and are capable of functioning both as acid and bases. When an ampholyte of the type NaHA is dissolved in water, it gives the following series of reactions

$$Na^+\,HA^- \xrightleftharpoons{H_2O} Na^+ + HA^-$$

$$HA^- + H_2O \rightleftharpoons A^{2-} + H_3O^+$$

$$HA^- + H_2O \rightleftharpoons H_2A + OH^-$$

$$2\,H_2O \rightleftharpoons H_3O^+ + OH^-$$

The total PBE for the system is

$$[H_3O^+] + [H_2A] = [OH^-] + [A^{2-}]$$

Substituting both $[H_2A]$ and $[A^{2-}]$ as a function of $[H_3O^+]$ yields,

$$\left[H_3O^+\right] = \frac{\left[H_3O^+\right]^2 C_s}{\left[H_3O^+\right]^2 + K_1\left[H_3O^+\right] + K_1 K_2}$$

$$= \frac{K_a}{\left[H_3O^+\right]} = \frac{K_1 K_2 C_s}{\left[H_3O^+\right]^2 + K_1\left[H_3O^+\right] + K_1 K_2}$$

This can be simplified into,

$$\left[H_3O^+\right] = \sqrt{\frac{K_1 K_2 C_s}{K_1 + C_s}}$$

in most cases $C_s \gg K_1$, the equation further simplified to,

$$[H_3O^+] = \sqrt{K_1 K_2}$$

In $[H_3O^+]$ becomes independent of the concentration of the salt. A special property of ampholytes is that the concentration of the species HA is max at the pH corresponding to $[H_3O^+] = \sqrt{K_1 K_2}$

When the simplest amino acid salt, glycine hydrochloride is dissolved in water, it acts as diprotic acid and ionizes as

$$^+NH_3\,CH_2\,COOH + H_2O \rightleftharpoons {}^+NH_3\,CH_2\,COO^- + H_3O^+$$

$$^+NH_3\,CH_2\,COO^- + H_2O \rightleftharpoons {}^+NH_2\,CH_2\,COO^- + H_3O^+$$

The form $_+NH_3CH_2COO^-$ is an ampholyte because it also can act as a weak base.

$$^+NH_3\,CH_2\,COO^- + H_2O \rightleftharpoons {}^+NH_3\,CH_2\,COOH + OH^-$$

This type of substances which carries both a charged acidic and a charged basic moiety on the same molecule is termed as a zwitter ion. Because 2 charges balance each other, the molecule acts essentially as a neutral molecule. The pH at which the zwitter ion concentration is maximum is known as the isoelectric point, which can be calculated from $[H_3O^+] = \sqrt{K_1 K_2}$.

7.5   Solutions Containing Only a Diprotic Acid

If a solution is made by adding a diprotic acid, H_2A to water to give a concentration C_a, the terms C_{ab} and C_b are zero. In almost all instances, the terms containing K_w can be dropped and after dividing through by $[H_3O^+]$, we obtain,

$$[H_3O^+]^3 + [H_3O^+]^2\,K_1 - [H_3O^+]\,(K_1\,C_a - K_1\,K_2) - 2K_1\,K_2\,C_a = 0$$

If $C_a \gg K_2$ as is usually true

$$[H_3O^+]^3 + [H_3O^+]^2\,K_1 - [H_3O^+]\,K_1\,C_a - 2K_1\,K_2\,C_a = 0$$

If $[H_3O^+]$ is much greater than $2K_2$, the term $2K_1K_2\,C_a$ can be dropped and dividing through by $[H_3O^+]$ yields the quadratic equation.

$$[H_3O^+]^2 + [H_3O^+]^2\,K_1 - K\,C_a = 0$$

The assumptions C_a is much greater than K_2 and $[H_3O^+]$ is much greater than $2K_2$ will be valid whenever K_2 is much less than K_1. It C_a is much greater than $[H_3O^+]$ this equations simplifies to the equation which was obtained for a solution containing a monoprotic weak acid.

7.6 Solutions Containing Only an Ampholyte

If an ampholyte HA^- is dissolved in water to give a solution with concentration C_{ab}, the terms C_a and C_b in equation are zero

$$[H_3O^+]^4 + [H_3O^+]^3 (K_1 + 2C_b + C_{ab}) + [H_3O^+]^2 [K_1 (C_b - C_a) +$$
$$K_1 K_2 - K_w] - [H_3O^+] [K_1 K_2 (2C_a + C_b) + K_1 K_w] - K_1 K_2 K_w = 0$$

For most systems of practical importance, the first, third and fifth terms of that equation are negligible when compared to second and fourth terms and the equation becomes

$$[H_3O^+] = \sqrt{\frac{K_1 K_2 C_{ab} + K_1 K_w}{K_1 + C_{ab}}}$$

The term $K_2 C_{ab}$ is generally much greater than K_w, and

$$[H_3O^+] = \sqrt{\frac{K_1 K_2 C_{ab}}{K_1 + C_{ab}}}$$

If the solution is concentrated enough that C_{ab} is much greater than K,

$$[H_3O^+] = \sqrt{K_1 K_2}$$

7.7 Solutions Containing Only a Diacidic Base

In general, the calculation for solutions containing weak bases are easier to handle by solving for $[OH^-]$ rather than $[H_3O^+]$. Any equation in terms of $[H_3O^+]$ and acidity constants can be converted into terms of $[OH^-]$ and basicity constants by substituting $[OH^-]$ for $[H_3O^+]$, K_{b1}, for K_1, K_{b2} for K_2, C_b for C_a. These substitutions are made into the above eq. $[H_3O^+]^4 = 0$. Further for a solution containing only a diacidic base C_a and C_b are zero, all terms containing K_w can be dropped. C_b is much greater than K_{b2} and $[OH^-]$ is much greater than $2 K_{b2}$. The following expression results,

$$[OH^-]^2 + [OH^-] K_{b1} - K_{b1} C_b = 0$$

If C_b is much greater than $[OH^-]$, the equation simplifies to

$$[OH^-] = \sqrt{K_{b1} C_b}$$

Use of a simplified equation $[OH^-] = \sqrt{K_{b1}C_b}$ gives an answer for $[OH^-]$ that has a relative error of 24% as compared with the correct answer given by equation. $[OH^-]^2 + [OH^-] K_{b1} - K_{b1} C_b = 0$.

It is absolutely essential that all assumptions made in the calculation of $[H_3O^+]$ or $[OH^-]$ be verified

7.8 Two Independent Acid-Base Pairs

Consider a solution containing 2 independent acid-base pairs.

$$HB_1 + H_2O \rightleftharpoons H_3O^+ + B_1^-$$

$$K_1 = \frac{[H_3O^+][B_1^-]}{[HB_1]}$$

$$HB_2 + H_2O \rightleftharpoons H_3O^+ + B_2^-$$

$$K_2 = \frac{[H_3O^+][B_2^-]}{[HB_2]}$$

A general equation for calculating the pH of this type of solution can be developed by considering a solution made by adding to water the acids HB_1 and HB_2 in concentrations C_{a1} and C_{a2} and the bases B_1^- and B_2^- in concentrations C_{b1} and C_{b2}. The PBE for this system is $[H_3O^+] + [HB_1]_{B_1} + [HB_2]_{B_2} = [OH^-] + [B_1^-]_{A1} + [B_2^-]_{A2}$ where the subscripts refer to the sources of the species in the PBE. Replacing these species concentration as a function of $[H_3O^+]$ gives

$$[H_3O^+] + \frac{[H_3O^+]C_{b1}}{[H_3O^+]+K_1} + \frac{[H_3O^+]C_{b2}}{[H_3O^+]+K_2} = \frac{K_w}{[H_3O^+]} + \frac{K_1 C_{a1}}{[H_3O^+]+K_2} + \frac{K_2 C_{a2}}{[H_3O^+]+K_2}$$

which can arranged to

$$[H_3O^+]^4 + [H_3O^+]^3 (K_1 + K_2 + C_{b1} + C_{b2}) + [H_3O^+] \times$$
$$[K_1 (C_{b2} - C_{a1}) + K_2 (C_{b1} - C_{b2}) + K_1 K_2 - K_w] -$$
$$[H_3O^+] (K_1 K_2 + C_{a1} + C_{a2}) + K_w (K_1 + K_2)] - K_1 K_2 K_w = 0$$

7.9 Solutions Containing 2 Weak Acids

In systems containing 2 weak acids, C_{b1} and C_{b2} are zero, and all terms in K_w can be ignored in above eq. For all systems of practical importance, C_{a1} and C_{a2} are much greater than K_1 and K_2 so the equation simplifies to

$$[H_3O^+]^2 + [H_3O^+] (K_1 + K_2) - (K_1 C_{a1} + K_2 C_{a2}) = 0$$

If C_{a1} and C_{a2} are both greater than $[H_3O^+]$ the equation simplifies to

$$\left[H_3O^+\right] = \sqrt{K_1\,C_{a1} + K_2\,C_{a2}}$$

7.10 Solutions Containing a Salt of a Weak Acid and a Weak Base

The salt of a weak acid and a weak base such as ammonium acetate, dissociates completely in aqueous solution to yield NH_4^+ and AC^-. The NH_4^+ is an acid and can be designated as HB_1 and the base AC^- can be designated as B_2^-. Since only a single Acid HB_1 and a single base B_2^- were added to water in concentration C_{a1} and C_{b2} respectively all other stichimetric concentration terms in $(H_3O^+)^2 + (H_3O^+)\,K_1 - K\,Ca = 0$ are zero. In addition, all terms containing K_w are negligibly small and may be dropped. Simplifying the eq. to

$$[H_3O^+]^2\,(K_1 + K_2 + C_{b2}) + [H_3O^+]\,[K_1\,(C_{b2} - C_{a1}) + K_1\,K_2] - K_1\,K_2\,C_{a1} = 0$$

In solutions containing a salt such as ammonium acetate, $C_{a1} = C_{b2} = C_s$. C_s is the concentration of salt added. In all systems of practical importance, $C_s \gg K_1$ or K_2 and above eq. can be simplified to

$$[H_3O^+]^2\,C_s + [H_3O^+]\,K_1K_2 - K_1\,K_2\,C_s = 0$$

which is a quadratic equation that can be solved in the usual manner. In most instances, however $C_s \gg [H_3O^+]$ and the quadratic equation reduces to

$$[H_3O^+] = \sqrt{K_1\,K_2} \qquad\qquad .....(7.39)$$

The K_1 and K_2 are not the successive acidity constants for a single diprotic acid system. K_1 is acidity constant for HB_1, and K_2 is acidity constant for conjugate acid HB_2 of the base B_2^-. The determination of $Acid_1$ and $Acid_2$ can be illustrated using ammonium acetate, and considering the acid and base added to the system interacting as follows.

$$\underset{Acid_1}{NH_4^+} + \underset{Base_2}{AC^-} \rightleftharpoons \underset{Acid_2}{HAC} + \underset{Base_1}{NH_3}$$

For this system K_1 is acidity constant for ammonium ion and K_2 is acidity constant for acetic acid.

When ammonium succinate is dissolved in water, it dissociates to yield $2\,NH_4^+$ cations and succinate (S^{2-}) anion.

These ions can enter into the following acid-base equilibrium

$$\underset{Acid_1}{NH_4^+} + \underset{Base_2}{S^{2-}} \rightleftharpoons \underset{Acid_2}{HS^-} + \underset{Base_1}{NH_3}$$

$$.....(7.40)$$

In this system $C_{b2} = C_s$ and $C_{a1} = 2\,C_s$ the concentration of salt added. If C_s is much greater than either K_1 or K_2 the eq. 7.40 can be simplified to

$$(H_3O^+)^2 - (H_3O^+)\,K_1 - 2K_1\,K_2 = 0$$

and if $\quad 2K_2 >> [H_3O^+],\ [H_3O^+]\,\sqrt{2\,K_1\,K_2}$

In this example, eq. 7.40 shows that K_1 is the acidity constant for the ammonium cation and K_2 referring to $Acid_2$, must be the acidity constant. For the bisuccinate species H^{S-} or the second acidity constant for succinic acid

In general, when $Acid_2$ comes from a poly protic acid H_nA, equation obtained is

$$[H_3O^+]^2 - [H_3O^+]\,K_1\,(n-1) - n\,K_1\,K_2 = 0 \qquad \text{and}$$

$$[H_3O^+] = \sqrt{n\,K_1\,K_2} \qquad\qquad .....(7.41)$$

In eq. 7.40 base was assumed to be monoprotic. This equation would not be valid for salts such as ammonium succinate or ammonium phosphate. The solution to these equations yields a pH value above the final pK_a for the system. Because the concentration of all species formed by the addition of more than one proton to an poly acidic base will be negligibly small and the assumption of only a proton addition becomes quite valid.

7.11 Solutions Containing a Weak Acid and a Weak Base

Up to now the acid and base were added in the form of a single salt. They can be added as 2 separate salts or an acid and a salt however forming buffer solutions. For example consider a solution made by dissolving equimolar amounts of sodium acid phosphate. NaH_2PO_4 and disodium citrate $Na_2\,H\,C_6H_5\,O_7$ in water. Both salts dissociate to give the amphoteric species $H_2PO_4^-$ and $H\,C_6\,H_5\,O_7^{2-}$ causing a problem in deciding which species to designate as HB_1 and which to designate as B_2^-. This problem can be resolved by considering the acidity constants for the 2 species in question. The acidity constant for $H_2PO_4^-$ is 7.2 and that for the species $H\,C_6\,H_5\,O_7^{2-}$ is 6.4. The citrate species being more acidic, acts as the acid in the following equilibrium.

$$\underset{Acid_1}{H\,C_6\,H_5\,O_7^{2-}} + \underset{Base_2}{H_2PO_4^-} \rightleftharpoons \underset{Acid_2}{H_3PO_4} + \underset{Base_1}{C_6\,H_5\,O_7^{3-}}$$

$$.....(7.44)$$

Thus K_1 in eq. 7.39 is K_3 for the citric acid system, and K_2 in eq. 7.39 is K_1 for the phosphoric acid system.

The equilibrium shown in eq. 7.42 illustrates the fact that the system made by dissolving $NaH_2\,PO_4$ and $Na_2\,H\,C_6\,H_5\,O_7$ in water is identical to that made by dissolving H_3PO_4 and $Na_3\,C_6\,H_5\,O_7$ in water. In the latter case, H_3PO_4 is HB_1 and the tricitrate is B_2^-

and if the 2 substances are dissolved in equimolar amounts eq. 7.39 is valid for the system.

A slightly different situation arises for equimolar combinations of substances such as succinic acid $H_2 C_4 H_4 O_4$ and tribasic sodium phosphate Na_3PO_4. In this case, it is obvious that succinic acid is the acid, which can protonate the base to yield the species $H C_4 H_4 O_4^-$ and $HP O_4^{2-}$. The acid succinate (pK_a 5.63) is a stronger acid than HPO_4^{2-} (pK_a 12) however, an equilibrium cannot be established between these species and the species originally added to water. Instead, the $HP O_4^{2-}$ is protonated by the acid succinate to give $C_4H_4O_4^{2-}$ and $H_2P O_4^-$. This is illustrated in the following

$$H_2 C_4 A_4 O_4 + P O_4^{3-} \rightarrow H C_4 H_4 O_4^- + H P O_4^{2-} \qquad \ldots\ldots(7.43)$$

$$\underset{\text{Acid}_1}{H C_4 H_4 O_4^-} + \underset{\text{Base}_2}{HPO_4^{2-}} \rightleftharpoons \underset{\text{Base}_1}{C_4 H_4 O_4^{2-}} + \underset{\text{Acid}_2}{H_2 PO_4^-} \qquad \ldots\ldots(7.44)$$

Thus K_1 in eq. 7.44 is K_2 for the succinic acid system and K_2 in eq. 7.39 is actually K_2 from the phosphoric acid system. Eqs. 7.43, 7.44 illustrate the fact that solutions made by dissolving equimolar amounts of $H_2 C_4 H_4 O_4$ and $Na_3 PO_4$, $Na H C_4 H_4 O_4$ and $Na_2 HO_4$ or $Na_2 C_4 H_4 O_4$ and $Na H_2 PO_4$ in water all equilibrate to same pH and are identical.

Acidity Constants

One of the most important properties of a drug molecule is its acidity constant, which for many drugs can be related to physiologic and pharmacologic activity, solubility, rate of solution. Extent of binding rate of absorption.

Effect of ionic strength on acidity constants

For example in a reaction

$$\underset{\text{Acid}_1}{HAC} + \underset{\text{Base}_2}{H_2O} \rightleftharpoons \underset{\text{Acid}_2}{H_3O^+} + \underset{\text{Base}_1}{AC^-}$$

ionization constant is replaced by acidity constant K_a

$$K_a = \frac{[H_3O^+][AC^-]}{[HAC]}$$

In dilute solutions of acetic acid, water is in sufficient excess to be regarded as constant at about 55.3 moles/lt.

For weak bases which are non ionized

$$B + H_2O \rightleftharpoons OH^- + BH^+$$

$$K_b = \frac{[OH^-][BH^+]}{[B]}$$

Here K_b is known as basicity constant.

Upton now, the solutions were considered dilute enough that the effect of ionic strength on the acid-base equilibria could be ignored. A more exact treatment for the ionization of a weak acid for example would be

$$HB + H_2O \rightleftharpoons H_3O^+ + B$$

$$K = \frac{a_{H_3O^+} \propto_B}{\propto_{HB}} = \frac{[H_3O^+][B]}{[HB]} \cdot \frac{\gamma H_3O^+ \cdot \gamma_B}{\gamma_{HB}} \qquad .....(7.45)$$

K is the thermodynamic acidity constant and the charges on the species have been omitted to make the equations more general. Eq. 7.45 illustrates the fact that in solving equation involving acidity constants both the concentration and the activity coefficient of each species must be considered. One way to simplify the problem would be to define the acidity constant as an apparent constant in terms of the hydronium ion activity and species concentration and activity coefficient as shown below.

$$K = a_{H_3O^+} \frac{[B]}{[HB]} \frac{\gamma_B}{\gamma_{HB}} = K' \frac{\gamma_B}{\gamma_{HB}}$$

Applying – log on both sides

$$K' = K \cdot \frac{\gamma_{HB}}{\gamma_B}$$

$$-\log K' = -\log K - \log \frac{\gamma_{HB}}{\gamma_B}$$

$$PK' = P^k + \log \frac{\gamma_B}{\gamma_{HB}} \qquad .....(7.46)$$

The following form of Debye-Huckel eq. can be used for ionic strength up to about 0.3μ.

$$-\log \gamma_i = \frac{0.51 z_i^2 \sqrt{\mu}}{1 + \propto B\sqrt{\mu}} - K_s \mu \qquad .....(7.47)$$

where z_i is the charge on the species 'I'. The value of the constant aB can be taken to be approximately 1 at 25 °C and K_s is a 'salting-out' constant. At moderate ionic strengths, K_s can be assumed to be approximately the same for both the acid and its conjugate base. Thus, for an acid with charge 'z' going to a base with charge $z - 1$.

$$p^{K'} = p^{K} + \frac{0.51(2z-1)\sqrt{\mu}}{1+\sqrt{\mu}}$$

If either the acid or its conjugate base is a zwitter ion, it will have a large dipole moment and the expression for its activity coefficient must contain a term K_r, the "salting-in" constant. Thus for zwitter ions [+–]

$$- \log r_{+1} = (K_r - K_s)\,\mu \qquad\qquad .....(7.48)$$

The first ionization of an amino acid such as glycine hydrochloride involves an acid with a charge of $+1$ going to the zwitter ion [+ –], combining eqns. 7.47, 7.48 with eq. 7.46 gives

$$P'_{k_1} = P_{K_1} + \frac{0.51\sqrt{\mu}}{1+\sqrt{\mu}} - K_r\mu \qquad\qquad .....(7.49)$$

The second ionization step involves the zwitter ion going to a species with a charge of -1. Thus using eqns. 7.47, 7.48, 7.49 gives,

$$P'_{k_2} = P_{K_2} + \frac{0.51\sqrt{\mu}}{1+\sqrt{\mu}} - K_r\mu \qquad\qquad .....(7.50)$$

The 'salting-in' constant, K_r, is approximately 0.32 for alpha-amino acids in water and approximately 0.6 for dipeptides. Use of these values for K_r enables eqs. 7.48, 7.50 to be used for solutions with ionic strengths up to about 0.3 μ.

The procedure to be used in solving pH problems in which the ionic strength of the solution must be considered is as follows.

(a) Convert all P^k values needed for the problem into $P^{k'}$ values.

(b) Solve the appropriate equations in the usual manner.

Free Energy of Ionization and the Effect of Temperature on Ionic Equilibria

The standard free energy change Δc_1^0 of a reaction is related to the equilibrium constant. Therefore the standard free energy change of an ionization reaction can be computed from ionization constant, K_a

$$\Delta c_1^0 = -\,RT \, ln \, K_a$$

using the Pk_a, we can write eq. 7.51 as

$$\Delta c_1^0 = 2.303\, RT\, PK_a$$

although Δc_1^0 is positive, it is not Δc_1^0 but rather Δ a that determines whether a process is spontaneous

$$\Delta c_1 = \Delta c_1^0 + RT\, l_n\, a$$

By writing above equation as

$$\Delta c_1 = RT\, ln\, \frac{Q}{K} \qquad .....(7.52)$$

Spontaneity of the reaction depend on the relative values of the quantities Q and K. If Q is smaller than K. signifying that the concentration of the products are below the values at equilibrium. Δc_1 will have a negative sign and the process will move spontaneously toward a stable of equilibrium. If Q is larger than K, the concentration of the products is greater than the equilibrium values, Δc_i will have a positive sign and the process will be nonspontaneous. If $K = a$, then $\Delta c_i = 0$ and the system is at equilibrium.

The positive value of Δc_1^0 signifies that the electrolyte in its standard state of unit activity cannot dissociate spontaneously into ions of unit activity. Ionization does occur, nevertheless, its possibility being shown by the sign of Δc_i and not by the sign of Δc_1^0. This fact was brought out in an example in which neither the reactant nor the products were in their standard states.

Standard Thermodynamic Values for Ionization of Acetic Acid

	CH_3COOH	**CH_3COO^-**	**H^+**
ΔH_f° (Kcal/mole)	−116.10	−116.16	0
$\Delta c_{i\,f}^\circ$ (Kcal/mole)	−94.8	−88.29	0
S° (cal/deg mole)	42.7	20.7	0

In the above values, f stands for free energy or enthalpy of formation S°-standard thermodynamic property as designated by superscript "o". ΔS is absolute entropy of a substance based on its entropy value above zero Kelvin. Now the change in enthalpy, entropy, and free energy in a reaction can be characterised by the standard enthalpy, entropy, free energy changes. $\Delta H^\circ f$, ΔS° and Δc_1^0 respectively. These are obtained by taking differences between the ΔH°_f, S° and $\Delta c_{1\,f}^0$ of the product and reactant.

In its standard state of 1μ aqueous solutions, the value of the hydrogen ion for these thermodynamic properties is 'o' as seen in above table.

Then standard enthalpy, entropy changes ΔH^o and ΔS^o for ionization reaction are the values for product CH_3COO^- minus the values for the reactant at 25 °C.

$$OH^o = (-116.16) - (-116.10) = -0.060 \text{ k cal/mole}$$

$$= -60.0 \text{ cal/mole}$$

$$\Delta S^o = 20.7 - 42.7 = -22.0 \text{ cal/deg mole}$$

Now from the equation $\Delta c_1^0 = 2.303 \text{ RT PK}_a$

$$p^{Ka} = + \Delta c_1^0 /(2.303) \text{ RT}$$

Because
$$\Delta c_1^0 = \Delta H^o - T\Delta s^o \qquad\qquad .....(7.53)$$

We also have
$$2.303 \log K_a = \frac{\Delta S^o}{R} - \frac{OH^o}{RT} \qquad\qquad .....(7.54)$$

Knowing ΔH^o_f and S^o simply having $\Delta C^0_{1\,f}$ for both reactants and products, we can obtain K_a and p^{Ka} for ionization of weak acids and weak bases. This procedure also used to calculate equilibrium constant for non ionic chemical reactions.

Continuing with acetic acid. Using eq. 7.54

$$2.303 \log K_a = \frac{-22.0}{1.9872} - \frac{-60}{(1.9872)(298.15)} = 10.96958$$

$$\log K_a = 4.763; K_a = 1.73 \times 10^{-5}$$

$$p^{Ka} = 4.76$$

	ΔH_f^o	S^o	Δc_{1f}^0
H_2CO_3 aqueous	−167.22	44.8	−148.94
HCO_3^- aqueous	−165.39	21.8	−140.26
CO_3^{2-} aqueous	−161.84	−13.6	−126.17

Here ΔH_f^o and Δc_{1f}^0 are heat and free energy of formation at 25 °C (298.15 k) respectively and S^o is the absolute entropy at 25 °C. The "o" indicates that these thermodynamic quantities are for each species in its standard state of 1 m aqueous solution at 1 atm 'P' and ordinary temperature.

The reaction for 1st stage is

$$H_2CO_3 \rightarrow HCO_3^- + H^+$$

and the standard enthalpy, entropy and free energy are respectively

$$\Delta H^\circ = \Delta H_f^\circ \ (HCO_3^- \ aq) - \Delta H_f^\circ \ (H_2CO_3)$$

$$= -(165.39) - (-167.22) = 1.830 \ kcal/mole$$

$$= 1830 \ cal/mole$$

$$\Delta S^\circ = S^\circ \left(HCO_3^-\right)_{aq} - S^\circ \left(H_2CO_3\right)$$

$$(21.8) - (44.8) = -23.0 \ cal/deg \ mole$$

$$\Delta c_1^0 = \Delta c_{1f}^0 \left(HCO_3^- \ aq\right) - \Delta c_{1f}^0 \left(H_2CO_3\right)$$

$$= (-140.26) - (-148.94) = 8.680 \ k \ cal/mole$$

$$= 8680 \ cal/mole$$

The ionization constant for 1st stage of ionization of H_2CO_3 is obtained from the equation

$$\Delta c_1^0 = \Delta H^\circ - T \ \Delta S^\circ = -RT \ ln \ K_1 \qquad or$$

$$ln \ K_1 = \frac{\Delta S_{12}^0}{R} - \frac{\Delta H_{12}^0}{RT} = \frac{\Delta c_{12}^0}{RT}$$

Substituting the values, from $H_2CO_3 \rightarrow HCO_3^- + H^+$ we obtain

$$ln \ K_1 = \frac{-23.0}{1.9872} - \frac{1830}{(1.9872)(298.15)}$$

$$= -14.663; \ log \ K_1 = ln \ K_1/2.303$$

$$- log \ K_1 = P \ K_1 = 6.32$$

Harned and Owen suggested an empirical equation by which ionization constant and temperature will be related.

$$log \ K = -\frac{A}{T} - CT + D \qquad\qquad .....(7.55)$$

where A, C, D are constant obtained by careful experimentation. Ionization constant of many of weak electrolytes pass through a maximum value between 0 °C and 60 °C and the temperature at which maximum ionization occurs is given by the expression

$$T_{max} = \sqrt{\frac{A}{C}}$$

The dissociation exponent at this temperature is

$$P^k \ T_{max} = 2\sqrt{AC} - D \qquad\qquad .....(7.56)$$

The thermodynamic quantities for ionization are also obtained by use of constant A, C, and D

$$\Delta c_1^0 = 2.3026\ R\ (A - DT + CT^2)$$

$$\Delta H^\circ = 2.3026\ R\ (A - CT^2)$$

$$\Delta S^\circ = 2.3026\ R\ (D - 2\ CT)$$

Thermodynamic Constants of Ionization

Electrolyte	A	C	D	T_{max} (k)	$P^K\ T_{max}$	Δc_1^0 25 °C cal/mole	ΔH° 25 °C cal/mole	ΔS° 25 °C cal/deg mole
Formic acid	1342.85	0.015168	5.2243	297.5	3.7519	5117	−23	−17.6
Acetic acid	1170.48	0.013399	3.1649	295.6	4.7555	6486	−92	−22.1
Propionic acid	1213.26	0.014.55	3.3860	293.8	4.8729	6647	−163	−22.8
Boric acid	2193.55	0.016499	3.0395	364.4	8.9923	12596	3.328	−31.1
Barbital	2324.47	0.011856	3.3491	-	-	-	-	-
Lactic acid	1304.72	0.014926	4.9639	-	-	-	-	-

In this chapter, we considered a process in which an electric current is produced by allowing a chemical reaction to occur. Such as electro chemical reaction depends on relative abilities of species in solution to be oxidised or reduced and this in turn is related to processes occurring at electrodes that connect the species in solution to any external circuit. The electro chemical reactions can be used to determine pH, activity coefficients or quantity of a specific ion in solution. These determinations involve potentiometry in which there is no significant current flow through the system.

Calculations

1. A quantity of HCl (1.5×10^{-3} μ) is added to water at 25 °C to increase the hydrogen ion concentration from 1×10^{-7} to 1.5×10^{-3} mol/lt. What is new hydroxyl ion concentration?

   As $\qquad \left[H_3O^+\right] \times \left[OH^-\right] = K_w \cong 1 \times 10^{-14}$ at 25 °C

   $$\left[OH^-\right] = \frac{K_w}{\left[H_3O^+\right]}$$

   $$= \frac{1 \times 10^{-14}}{1.5 \times 10^{-3}} = 6.7 \times 10^{-12}\ \text{mole/lt.}$$

2. Ammonia has a K_b of 1.74×10^{-5} at 25 °C. Calculate K_a for its conjugate acid NH_4^+.

$$K_w = K_a \times K_b$$

$$K_a = \frac{K_w}{K_b}$$

$$= \frac{1.00 \times 10^{-14}}{1.74 \times 10^{-5}}$$

$$K_a = 5.75 \times 10^{-10}$$

3. If the pH of the solution is 5.72, what is hydronium ion concentration?

$$pH = -\log [H_3O^+] = 5.72$$

$$\log [H_3O^+] = -5.72 = -6 + 0.28$$

$$[H_3O^+] = \text{antilog } 0.28 \times \text{antilog } (-6)$$

$$[H_3O^+] = 1.91 \times 10^{-6} \text{ mole/lt}$$

4. The dissociation constant of acetic acid is 1.75×10^{-5} at 25 °C. Calculate its pKa value.

$$K_a = 1.75 \times 10^{-5}$$

$$\log K_a = \log 1.75 + \log 10^{-5}$$

$$= 0.2430 - 5 = -4.757 \text{ or } -4.76$$

$$pK_a = -\log K_a$$

$$= -(4.76) = 4.76$$

5. Calculate pH of 0.01 μ solution of salycilic acid which has a K_a value of 1.06×10^{-3} at 25 °C.

Using $[H_3O^+] = \sqrt{K_a C_a}$

$$[H_3O^+] = \sqrt{(1.06 \times 10^{-3}) \times (1.0 \times 10^{-2})}$$

$$= 3.26 \times 10^{-3} \text{ M}$$

The approximation that $C_a \gg H_3O^+$ is not valid by using equation

$$[H_3O^+] = \frac{-K_a + \sqrt{K_a^2 + 4 K_a C_a}}{2}$$

$$[H_3O^+] = -\frac{(1.06\times10^{-3})}{2} \times \frac{\sqrt{(1.06\times10^{-3})^2 + 4(1.06\times10^{-3})(1.0\times10^{-2})}}{2}$$

$$= 2.77 \times 10^{-3} \; \mu$$

$$pH = -\log(2.77 \times 10^{-3}) = 2.56$$

(b) What is pH of a solution containing acetic acid 0.5 μ and sodium acetate 0.05 μ;

$$[H_3O^+] = \frac{K_a \, C_a}{C_b}$$

$$= \frac{(1.75\times10^{-5})\times 0.5}{5\times10^{-2}}$$

$$= 1.75 \times 10^{-4} \; \mu$$

$$pH = -\log[H_3O^+]$$

$$= -\log(1.75 \times 10^{-4}) = 3.756$$

7. Calculate pH of a 5×10^{-3} μ solution of sodium bicarbonate at 25 $^{\circ}$C. The acidity constants for carbonic acid are $K_1 = 4.6 \times 10^{-7}$ and $K_2 = 4.8 \times 10^{-11}$.

$$[H_3O^+] = \sqrt{K_1 \, K_2}$$

$$[H_3O^+] = \sqrt{(4.6\times10^{-7})\times(4.8\times10^{-11})}$$

$$= 4.7 \times 10^{-9} \; \mu$$

$$pH = -\log(4.7 \times 10^{-9})$$

$$= 8.32$$

8. Calculate pH of a 0.01 μ solution of ammonium acetate. The acidity constant for acetic acid is $K_2 = K_a = 1.39 \times 10^{-5}$ and the basicity constant for ammonia is $K_b = 1.34 \times 10^{-5}$.

K_1 can be found by dividing K_b for ammonia into K_w

$$K_1 = \frac{1\times10^{-14}}{1.34\times10^{-5}} = 7.46\times10^{-10}$$

$$H_3O^+ = \sqrt{(7.46\times10^{-10})\times(1.39\times10^{-5})}$$

$$= 1.018 \times10^{-7}$$

$$pH = -\log(1.018 \times 10^{-7})$$

$$pH = 6.992$$

9. Calculate pH of a solution containing succinic acid and tribase sodium phosphate each at a concentration of 0.01m. The second acidity constant for the succinic acid is 4.6×10^{-6}. The second acidity constant for the phosphoric acid is 5.2×10^{-8}.

$$pH = \frac{1}{2}\left(pK_1 + pK_2\right)$$

$$= \frac{1}{2}\left(-\log\left(4.6 \times 10^{-6}\right) + \left[-\log\left(5.2 \times 10^{-8}\right)\right]\right)$$

$$= \frac{1}{2}\left(5.33 + 7.28\right)$$

$$= \frac{1}{2}\left(12.61\right)$$

$$pH = 6.305$$

10. Calculate pH of a 0.01 μ solution of acetic acid to which enough KCl had been added to give an ionic strength of 0.01 μ at 25 °C. The pK_a for acetic acid is 5.84.

(a)
$$pK_a' = 5.84 - \frac{0.51\sqrt{0.10}}{1 + \sqrt{0.10}}$$

$$= 5.84 - 0.12 = 5.72$$

(b) Taking $\log pH = \frac{1}{2}\left(pK_a' - \log C_a\right)$

Here pK_a' is pKa

$$pH = \frac{1}{2}\,(5.72 + 2) = 3.86$$

11. Calculate pH of 10^{-3} m solution of glycine at an ionic strength of 0.10 at 25 °C. The pK_a values for glycine are $pK_1 = 3.31$ and $pK_2 = 10.64$.

(a)
$$pK_1' = 3.31 + \frac{0.51\sqrt{0.10}}{1 + \sqrt{0.10}} - 0.32\,(0.10)$$

$$= 3.31 + 0.12 - 0.03 = 3.4$$

(b)
$$pK_2' = 10.64 - \frac{0.51\sqrt{0.10}}{1 + \sqrt{0.10}} + 0.32\,(0.10)$$

$$= 10.64 - 0.12 + 0.03 = 10.55$$

(c)   Taking an equation $\text{pH} = \dfrac{1}{2}\left(p^{K_1} + p^{K_2}\right)$

$$= \dfrac{1}{2}\left(3.4 + 10.55\right)$$

$$\text{pH} = 6.975$$

12. pK_a value for weak acid amobarbital at 25 °C is 7.96. Calculation the standard free energy change for ionization of this barbituric derivative.

$$\Delta c_1^0 = 2.303 \times RT \times pKa$$

$$= 2.303 \times 1.9872 \times 298 \times 7.96$$

$$= 10{,}855.9 \text{ cal/mole}$$

$$\Delta c_1^0 = 10.86 \text{ kcal/mole}$$

7.12 Questions

1. What are Isosmotic, Isotonic, hypertonic and hypotonic solution. Discuss the various methods available for adjustment of tonicity of solutions.

2. Define Osmosis, Osmotic pressure and describe the measurement of osmotic pressure by Berkeley and Hartly's method.

3. Define and describe the following.

   (i)   Buffers

   (ii) Buffer capacity

CHAPTER 8

ELECTROCHEMISTRY

8.1 Introduction

Electrochemistry deals with the:

1. use of electrical energy for the dissociation of chemical compound (electrolysis),
2. use of chemical reactions for the production of electrical energy (electrochemical cells) and
3. use of electrical energy in the study and preparation of chemical substances.

Electric current is considered in general as flow of electric charges through the conducting medium. This conducting medium is referred to as "Electric Conductor". E.g., solid metals, fused metals, salts (or) aqueous solutions.

Definition: The substance which allows the electric current to flow through it is called electric conductor.

Electric conductors are of two types. They are:

1. Metallic conductors (or) electronic conductors (solids)
2. Electrolytic conductors

1. ***Metallic Conductors:*** In these conductors, flow of electric current is due to the movement of free electrons from high negative potential region to a lower

positive potential region without producing any chemical changes in the conductor.

E.g. Cu, Ag, Al, Cds, CuS etc.

2. ***Electrolytic Conductors:*** In these conductors, the flow of current is due to the migration of ions towards oppositely charged electrodes producing chemical changes in the conductor.

E.g. KCl, NaCl, K_2SO_4, HCl, HNO_3, NaOH, KOH etc

These are generally referred as electrolytes.

When a chemical reaction occurs, electric current is produced due to the flow of electrons. These electrons are consumed by electrodes that are present in an electrochemical cell. The chemical reaction depends upon the relative abilities of the ions or the substances that are present in the solution i.e., oxidation or reduction.

8.1.1 Electrochemical Cells

They are also known as galvanic cells or electrical cells or chemical cells or voltaic cell.

Definition: It is a device which uses a spontaneous redox reaction for the generation of electrical energy.

Electrochemical cell consists of two compartments. The two compartments are separated by porous diaphragm. Each compartment is referred to as half-cell. Porous diaphragm allows the electric contact between the solutions but does not permit excessive mixing of two solutions. The electrodes are placed in the respective compartments namely in the right half-cell and in the left half-cell. The anode is placed in left-half cell and cathode is placed in right-half cell containing electrolytes. Zinc electrode which acts as anode is placed in zinc sulphate solution in the left-half cell. The copper electrode is placed in copper sulphate solution which acts as cathode. An external wire is connected to two half-cells possessing electrodes and when the wires are joined a spontaneous reaction is occurred. The reaction observed at left-half cell is:

Anode reaction (oxidation)

$$Zn = Zn^{2+} + 2e^- \rightarrow E \text{ left} \qquad\qquad .....(8.1)$$

At right-half-cell is:

Cathode reaction (Reduction)

$$Cu^{+2} + 2e^- \rightarrow Cu \rightarrow E \text{ right} \qquad\qquad .....(8.2)$$

Zinc has a greater tendency to ionise. i.e., to lose electron. These electrons are released by zinc atoms and they pass into the solution. The extent of release of electrons depends upon the electro negativity and the concentration of the metal ions. Lower the electro negativity of the metal, greater is the tendency to release the electron.

The electrons pass from this negatively charged electrode to the copper electrode through external copper wire.

And at cathodes, copper ions from the solution take on electron and deposit the copper atoms on the surface of the electrode. The cathode thus loses the electron and is considered to be positively charged. This spontaneous reaction represents the oxidation of zinc metal at the zinc electrode and copper ions are reduced at the copper electrode.

In order to obtain the over all cell reaction, the two cell reactions must be added and is represented as:

$$E_{Left} \rightarrow \quad Zn \rightarrow Zn^{2+} + 2e^- \qquad\qquad .....(8.3)$$

$$E_{Right} \rightarrow \quad Cu^{2+} + 2e^- \rightarrow Cu \qquad\qquad .....(8.4)$$

$$Zn + Cu^{2+} \rightarrow Zn^{2+} + Cu \rightarrow over\ all\ reaction \qquad .....(8.5)$$

$$E_{cell} = E_{left} + E_{right}$$

The individual electrode potential occurs at the junction between each electrode and its surrounding solution. The sum of the two electrodes refers to the E_{cell} which represents EMF or voltage of cell. There is a large difference between the emf and the potential of the cell. EMF refers to the complete voltage of the cell and potential refers to the voltage of the electrode.

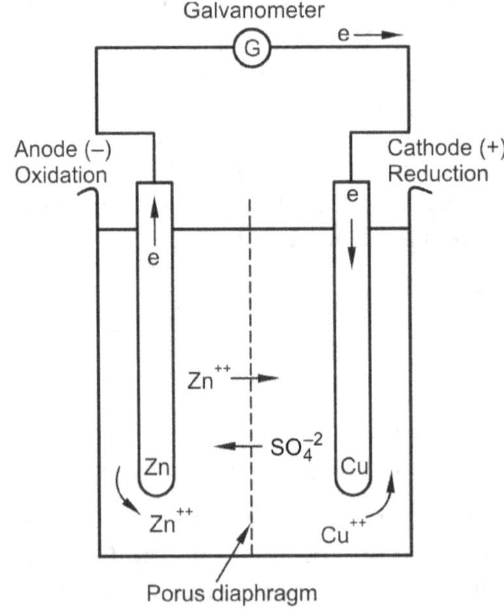

Fig. 8.1 Electrochemical cell.

8.1.2 Half Reactions

Let us consider the reaction,

$$2Na + Cl_2 \rightarrow 2Na^+ + Cl^-$$

This reaction takes place by transfer of electron from sodium to chlorine. Sodium loses an electron and is said to be oxidised and gets converted to Na^+ ion. This electron is gained by the chlorine atom and is reduced to chloride ion. This reaction which occurs about by loss of electron (oxidation) and gain of electron (reduction) simultaneously is called an oxidation reduction reaction or redox reaction. In the redox reaction no free electrons are generated.

The redox reaction is considered as a combination of two reactions.

For example:
$$2Na \rightarrow 2Na^+ + 2e^- \qquad \text{(oxidation)} \qquad\qquad .....(8.6)$$
$$Cl_2 + 2e^- \rightarrow 2Cl^- \qquad \text{(Reduction)} \qquad\qquad .....(8.7)$$

$$2Na + Cl_2 \rightarrow 2Na^+ + Cl^- \qquad\qquad\qquad .....(8.8)$$

These are the reactions of the half components, they are called half-reaction. The first half-reaction that proceeds by oxidation is referred to as oxidised-half reaction and that proceeds by reduction is called reduction-half reaction.

When these two reductions are added, it gives the net redox reaction.

One may have a doubt that how a redox reaction is able to produce an electric current. This can be explained by taking example.

Consider a zinc has dipped in copper-sulphate solution and copper metal is deposited on the zinc bar by the replacement of zinc.

The net reaction is

$$Zn + Cu^{+2} \rightarrow Zn^{+2} + Cu \qquad\qquad .....(8.9)$$

It is a redox reaction and the Half reactions include in it are:
$$Zn \rightarrow Zn^{+2} + 2e^- \qquad\qquad .....(8.10)$$
$$Cu^{+2} + 2e^- \rightarrow Cu \qquad\qquad .....(8.11)$$

In this, Zn is oxidised to give Zn^{+2} ions and Cu^{+2} ions are reduced to Cu atoms. The electrons released in the 1st half-reaction are used by the 2nd half-reaction. Both the half-reactions occur on the zinc bar itself; there is net change.

Consider the two half reactions occur in two separate compartments which are connected by a wire and the electrons which are produced in the left compartment flows to the other compartment through this wire. The flow of current will flow for instant and stop and is mainly due to: (i) the charge build up. (ii) the electron reaction from the left compartment and becomes positively charged and these electrons are received by right compartment and becomes negatively charged. Factors (i) and (ii) oppose the flow of electrons and this problem can be easily solved by using a salt-bridge. This is a U-filtered tube filled with an electrolyte such as NaCl, KCl and K_2SO_4 which provides the passage of ions from one compartment to the other compartment without mixing of the two ions. Due to this, ions will flow and the circuit is said to be completed and the electrons pass freely through the external wire by which are produced due to the redox reaction making the charge zero in the two compartments.

Applications: This electrochemical cell is used in the production of electrical energy which was produced due to chemical reaction and it was utilised by various industries, for domestic purpose.

- They are mainly used for quantitative analysis for the estimation of pH, determination of activity coefficients, solubility of substances in solutions.
- This is also used in plating technique on various ornaments, vessels (to avoid corrosion) etc., to gain appearance.

8.1.3 Cell Terminology

Current: The flow of electrons through a wire or any conductor.

Electrode: It is the material a metallic rod/bar/strip which conducts electrons into and out of a solution.

Anode: It is the electrode at which oxidation occurs and sends electrons into the outer circuit and posses negative charge shown as negative in cell diagrams.

Cathode: It is the electrode at which electrons are received from the outer circuit and has positive charge and shown as positive in cell diagrams.

Electrolyte: It is the salt solution in a cell.

Anode Compartment: It is the compartment of the cell in which the oxidation half-reaction occurs. It contains anode.

Cathode Compartment: It is the compartments, of the cell in which the reduction half-reaction occurs. It contains cathode.

Half-Cell: Each half- cell of an electrochemical cell, where oxidation occurs and the half where reduction occurs is called the half-cell.

Cell-Reaction: The flow of electrons from one electrode to the other electrode in an electrochemical cell is mainly occurred due to the half-reaction taking place in the anode and cathode compartments. The net chemical change obtained by the addition of two half-reactions is called the cell-reaction.

Example: (a) half-reactions $Zn(s) \rightarrow Zn^{2+}(aq) + 2e^-$ .....(8.12)

$$Cu^{2+}(aq) + 2e^- \rightarrow Cu(s) \qquad .....(8.13)$$

(b) Cell reaction is obtained by adding up the two half- reactions

$$Zn(s) + Cu^{+2}(aq) \rightarrow Zn^{+2}(aq) + Cu(s) \qquad .....(8.14)$$

8.1.4 Cell Potential or EMF

Consider a Zn-Cu voltaic cell. Electrons are released at anode and it becomes negatively charged. The negative electrode pushes the electrons through the external circuit by electrical repulsions. The copper electrode gets positive charge due to discharge of Cu^{+2} ions i.e., electrons from external circuit come and attract this electrode. The flow of current through the circuit is determined by the push of electrons at the anode and 'attraction' of electrons at the cathode. These two forces constitute the driving force or electrical pressure. This driving force is called electro motive force (EMF) or cell potential. It is measured in volts (v). It is also called as cell voltage.

A cell-diagram can be represented symbolically and for this consider a cell consists of two half-cells. Each half-cell is made of metal electrode contact with metal ion in the solution.

IUPAC Conventions: Cell diagram should be represented according to IUPAC conventions. The following are the conventions that are given by IUPAC.

1. Electrodes of the cell are always written that anode is on the left hand side and cathode is on the right hand side.

2. A single vertical line represents the junction between two different phases.

3. A double vertical line indicates the liquid junction or salt bridge or porous diaphragm i.e., electric contact between the two electrolyte solutions.

4. Half cell reaction taking place above the hydrogen electrode is the reduction reaction and below the hydrogen electrode is the oxidation reaction.

5. The half-cell which represents the oxidation takes place in the left and the reduction takes place in the right.

6. The reduction reaction is written in the order, ion and electrode and the oxidation reaction is in the order electrode and ion.

7. The symbol for an inert electrode like platinum is enclosed in bracket.

8. The emf of the cell is written on the right side of the cell diagram.

9. The electrode must be selected in such a way that the value of E° is positive making the reaction spontaneous.

10. If E° value is negative, the cell reaction would not be possible.

11. The higher the E° value, more will be the feasibility of the reaction.

12. The concentrations are also represented in the cell reaction.

    Example:

    1. zn $| Zn^{2+}(Zn^{2+}) \| Cu^{2+}(CCu^{2+})Cu$
           Oxidation   Reduction

       $|$ – Single vertical line represents junction between two phases

       $\|$ – Double vertical line represents a liquid junction or salt bridge that is an electric contact between two electrolyte solutions.

    2. $Mg | Mg^{2+} \| H^{+} | H_2$ (Pt) ← inert electrode.

    3. $Zn | ZnSO_4 \| CuSO_4 | Cu : e = + 1{\cdot}1$ V

Reversible Cell: A reversible cell is one when an external current is applied opposite to and infinitesimally greater than that of cell, causes the reverse function of electrochemical cell.

They are used to produce electrical energy from a chemical reaction. The hydrogen gas is not liberated.

E.g. Daniel cell which is composed of two electrodes i.e., Zinc immersed in $ZnSO_4$ solution and copper electrode immersed in $CuSO_4$ solution. The emf is about 1.1 volt.

The cell reaction is

$$Zn + Cu^{2+} \rightarrow Zn^{2+} + Cu \qquad\qquad .....(8.15)$$

The external EMF 1.1 volts is applied. The cell reaction is stopped and when an infinitesimally EMF greater than 1.1 volts is applied. The cell reaction is reversed (Zn^{2+} + Cu → Zn + Cu^{2+}) and if that EMFis removed then it returns to its original state.

Irreversible cell: It is a cell whose function cannot be reversed when an external current opposite to and infinitesimally EMF greater than cell is applied.

An irreversible cell cannot be converted into reversible cell. They cannot be used in the production of electrical energy. In the case of reversible cells, H_2 gas is produced.

e.g., Consider a cell composed of zinc and silver electrodes immersed in a solution of sulphuric acid. When two electrodes are connected, the following reaction occurs.

$$Zn + 2H^{+} \longrightarrow Zn^{+2} + H_2 \text{ (g)} \qquad\qquad .....(8.16)$$

If a greater EMF is applied by using external source, silver dissolves at one electrode and hydrogen evolves at other end. The cell reaction is :

$$2\, Ag \text{ (s)} + 2H^{+} \longrightarrow 2\, Ag^{+} + H_2 \text{ (g)} \qquad\qquad .....(8.17)$$

The reaction is not reversed and therefore not used in electro chemical reactions.

8.2 Calculating the EMF of a Cell

The EMF of a cell can be calculated from the half-cell potentials by using the formula.

$$E_{cell} = E_{cathoede} - E_{anode}$$

$$= ER - Eh$$

Where ER $\rightarrow$ Reduction potential of the right hand electrode

EL $\rightarrow$ Reduction potential of the left-hand electrode

Absolute values of the reduction potentials cannot be determined. The absolute value can be determined by connecting the half-cell with a standard hydrogen electrode whose reduction potential is zero.

e.g.: The individual electrode potentials of Zn – Ag electrodes are given as 0.80 and – 0. 763. Find out the E° of the cell.

Solution: The EMF of the cell can be calculated by using the formula:

$$E_{cell} = E_{right} - E_{left}$$

The cell reaction is : $Zn\ (s)\ |\ Zn^{+2}\ (aq)\ ||\ Ag^{+}\ (aq)\ |\ Ag$

$$E = E_{R} - E_{L}$$

$$= 0.80 - (- 0.763)$$

$$= 0.80 + 0.763$$

$$= 1.563\ V$$

8.2.1 Measurement of EMF of a Cell

The EMF of an unknown cell can be measured with the help of a potentiometer. A voltmeter draws a measurable amount of current from the circuit but a potentiometer measures by opposing the EMF of a cell with an applied potential. It simply balances one current flow against another without producing changes in potential due to cell resistance.

The principle that is involved in the potentiometer is Ohm's law. According to Ohm's law, the voltage is proportional to the resistance of the current flow

$$E = IR$$

It consists of a wire 'AB' which is about 1 metre long. The two ends of the wire are connected to a battery, B. Between the 0 and voltage divider a voltmeter is connected. The cell Ex is connected to the point '0' and the other end of the wire is connected to a contact 'x' which is movable through the press key and the galvanometer. The battery B is attached to a 16 metre long slide wire (00') of uniform diameter and possessing high resistance.

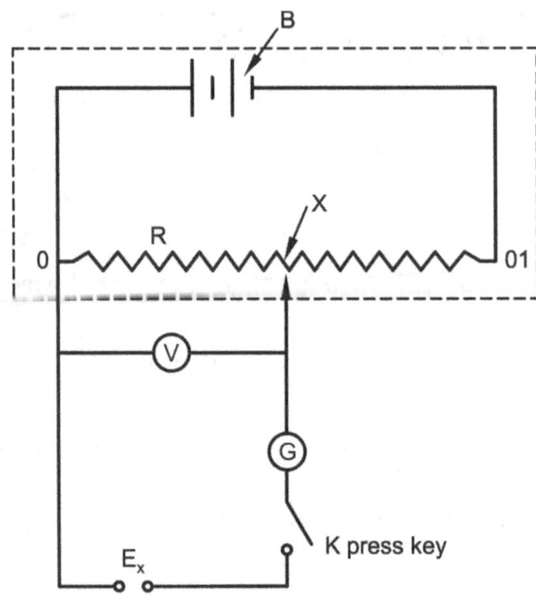

Fig. 8.2 Schematic diagram of potentiometer.

Working: When the key is pressed, the current will flow from the battery B, through a variable resistor R and to a Galvanometer 'G'. This variable resistor is also called voltage divider. The voltage divider is adjusted such that the galvanometer 'G' shows no deflection. When this occurs, the voltage read on the voltmeter v which is obtained from applied potential must be equal and it should be exactly opposite to the potential of the cell. This potential refers to the EMF of the cell being determined. The potential difference across the points 0-X on the resistor must be equal and opposite in sign to the EMF of the cell Ex.

The galvanometer is balanced quickly by tapping the key 'K' and the current does not flow for an appreciable period of time and during this when there is a deflection of G, the EMF measured for the cell can be considered a true equilibrium value. This method is sometimes referred to as Null-point potentiometry.

Applications: It is used in the determination of:

   (a)   Free energy change for the cell reaction.

   (b)   Degree of hydrolysis of salts in solution

   (c)   pH of the solutions

   (d)   Activity coefficients or concentrations of cells.

   (e)   Solubility of drugs.

           It also involved in determination of potentio metric titrations.

8.2.2 Single Electrode Potential

An electro-chemical cell consists of two half cells containing electrodes in it and dipping in their respective electrolyte solutions. The metal electrode transfers its ions into the solution. The individual electrode then develops a potential with respect to the solution. This potential is referred to as single electrode potential. The amount of the charge produced on individual electrode determines its single electrode potential.

The single electrode potential of a half cell depends upon:

   (a) concentration of ions in the solution,

   (b) tendency to form ions

   (c) the temperature.

   e.g.: In a Daniel cell in which the electrodes are not connected externally, the anode Zn/Zn^{2+} develops a negative charge and at cathode Cu/Cu^{2+} a positive charge is developed.

8.2.3 Standard EMF of a Cell

The EMF is represented by the symbol 'E' and it can be measured with help of a potentiometer. The value of EMF varies with the concentration of the reactants and the temperature of the cell. The standard EMF of a cell can be determined by maintaining the standard conditions such as:

   (a)   One molar solutions of reactants and products

   (b)   The temperature at 25°C.

Definition: The EMF of a cell with 1 molar solutions of reactants and products in a solution measured at 25 °C.

Standard EMF of a cell is represented by E^0. When gases are used instead of concentration of cell a pressure at 1 atm can be taken as a standard.

e.g.: Consider a Cu-Zn voltaic cell. The standard EMF of a cell is 1.10 V. It indicates that the EMF of a cell is measured by considering 1 molar solutions concentration of reactants and products and at 25 °C.

Cell Reaction: $Zn\,|Zn^{+2}$ (aq. 1M) $\|$ cu^{+2} (aq. 1M) $|\,Cu$ $E^0 = 1.1$ volts.

8.2.4 Determination of EMF of a Half Cell

The EMF of a cell can be determined by connecting them to voltmeter. There is no way of measuring the cell EMF directly. The convenient procedure is to measure the emf of the half cell by combining it with standard half-cell. The EMF of the newly constructed cell, E is determined with voltmeter EMF of the unknown cell E can be calculated by using

$$E_{measured} = E_R - E_L$$

If the standard Half-cell acts as anode, then equation becomes

$$E_R = E_{measured}$$

If the standard half-cell is cathode, the equation becomes

$$E_L = E_{measured}$$

(SHE) Standard hydrogen electrode is combined with another unknown half-cell in which they are connected to a voltmeter which gives EMF of the complete cell. The EMF of the cell is the EMF of the half cell.

For e.g.: Find out the EMF of a zinc electrode when it is combined with the SHE as the reference electrode. The EMF of the electro chemical cell is + 0.76 v.

Solution:
$$E_{cell} = E_R - E_L$$
$$0.76 = 0 - E_L^0$$
$$E_L = - 0.76 \text{ V}$$

i.e., EMF of the standard hydrogen electrode is arbitrarily fixed to zero. SHE should not take always as a cathode but sometimes it also acts as an anode. The electrodes should be taken as cathode and anode based upon the flow of electrons into or out of the solution.

But when we consider copper electrode in the place of zinc electrode, copper electrode acts as cathode i.e., SHE acts as anode.

When the zinc electrode is placed on the right half cell, the hydrogen electrode reaction is represented as :

$$2H^+ + 2e^- \rightarrow H_2 \qquad\qquad .....(8.18)$$

The electron flow from SHE and hence it acts as cathode. When the SHE is placed on the left half-cell, the containing copper electrode in right half-cell, the H_2 electrode reaction is represented as:

$$H_2 \rightarrow 2H^+ + 2e^- \qquad\qquad ..... (8.19)$$

The electron flow from copper SHE to copper electrode and hence it acts as anode.

IUPAC makes the SHE should always placed on the left-hand side i.e., electron flow from left to right and the other half-cell electrode gains the electron and becomes reduced and the measured EMF of the half-cell is the standard reduction potentials (SRP) or standard potentials.

If SHE is placed on the right-hand side, the potential obtained is standard oxidation potential (SOP).

According to IUPAC conventions, the SRP's are alone are the standard potentials.

8.3 Electrochemical Series

The standard reduction potentials of different electrodes are arranged in the order of decreasing potentials is known as electrochemical series.

It helps in finding out the reducing or oxidising ability of an electrode.

The electrodes which are +vely charged indicate that the reduction reaction involving addition of electron

$$M^+ + e^- \rightarrow \qquad M \qquad \rightarrow \qquad\qquad ..... (8.20)$$

The electrode which are –vely charged indicate that the oxidation reaction involving loss of electron

$$M \qquad \rightarrow \qquad M^+ + e^- \qquad\qquad ..... (8.21)$$

Also follows that the system with higher electrode potential will be reduced by the system with lower electrode potential.

Electrochemical Series

Reduction Reaction	Reduction Electrode	E^0 (Vol t)
$(1/2)\ Cl_2 + e^- = Cl^-$	$Cl^-|Cl_2$; Pt	$+1.360$
$(1/4)\ O_2 + H^+ + e^- = (1/2)\ H_2O$	$H^+|O_2$; Pt	$+1.229$
$Hg^{2+} + e^- = (1/2)\ Hg_2^{+2}$	$Hg^{+2}.Hg_2^{2+}.|$ Pt	$+0.907$
$Ag^+ + e^- = Ag$	$Ag^+|Ag$	$+0.799$
$(1/2)\ Hg^{2+}\ e^- = Hg$	$Hg_2^{2+}\ |$ Hg	$+0.789$
$Fe^{3+} + e^- = Fe^{2+}$	$Fe^{3+}, Fe^{2+}|$ Pt	$+0.771$
$(1/2)\ I_2 + e^- = I^-$	$I^-\ |\ I_2$	$+0.536$
$Fe(CN)_6^{3-} + e^- = Fe\ (CN)_6^{4-}$	$Fe(CN)_6^{3-}, Fe\ (CN)_6^{4-}\ |$ Pt	$+0.356$
$(1/2)\ Cu^{2+} + e^- = (1/2)\ Cu$	$Cu^{+2}|Cu$	$+0.337$
$(1/2)\ Hg_2\ Cl_2 + e^- = Hg + Cl$	$Cl\ |Hg_2|Cl_2,$ Hg	$+0.268$
$AgCl + e^- = Ag + Cl^-$	$Cl^-/Ag|Cl,$ Ag	$+0.223$
$AgBr + e^- = Ag + Br^-$	$Br^-|Ag\ Br,$ Ag	$+0.071$
$H^+ + e^- = (1/2)\ H_2$	$H^+|H_2,$ Pt	0.000
$(1/2)\ Pb^{2+} + e^- = (1/2)\ Pb$	$Pb^{+2}|Pb$	-0.126
$Ag\ I + e^- = Ag + I^-$	$I^-|AgI,$ Ag	-0.156
$(1/2)\ Ni^{2+} + e^- = (1/2)\ Ni$	$Ni^{2+}|Ni$	-0.230
$(1/2)\ Cd^{2+} + e^- = (1/2)\ Cd$	$Cd^{2+}|Cd$	-0.403
$(1/2)\ Fe^{2+} + e^- = (1/2)\ Fe$	$Fe^{2+}|Fe$	-0.490

$(1/2)\ Zn^{2+} + e^- = (1/2)\ Zn$	$Zn^{2+}|Zn$	-0.763
$Na^+ + e^- = Na$	$Na^+|Na$	-2.715
$K^+ + e^- = K$	$K^+|K$	-2.925
$Li^+ + e^- = Li$	$Li^+|Li$	-3.045

Consider a series of elements Cu, H_2, Ni, Zn and their ions. They act as reducing agents. The ions Cu^{2+}, H^+, Ni^{2+} ad Zn^{2+} act as electron acceptors. Electrodes are placed in a descending order i.e., placing the oxidising agents in descending order of their ability to attract the electron.

$$
\begin{array}{lccccl}
 & Cu^{2+} + 2e^- & \rightarrow & Cu & & E^0 = +0.34 \text{ v} \\
\text{Strength as} & 2H^+ + 2e^- & \rightarrow & H_2 & \text{Strength as} & E^0 = 0.00 \text{ v} \\
\text{oxidising agent} & Ni^{2+} + 2e^- & \rightarrow & Ni & \text{reducing agent} & E^0 = -0.25 \text{ v} \\
 & Zn^{2+} + 2e^- & \rightarrow & Zn & & E^0 = -0.76 \text{ v}
\end{array}
$$

E^0 becomes more negative down the series. This means that Cu^{+2} is the best oxidising agent i.e., Cu^{2+} shows the greatest tendency to be reduced. Conversely Zn^{2+} is the oxidising agent as it is a least electron attracting ion. Of these elements Cu, H_2, Ni and Zn, Zn is the best reducing agent, since E^0 for the half reaction is

$$Zn \rightarrow Zn^{2+} + e^- \qquad E^0 = +0.76 \text{ V} \qquad \dots\dots(8.22)$$

From the electro chemical series, it should be noted that:

1. The more positive the value of E^0, the better is the oxidising ability of the ion or compound on moving upward,
2. The more is the value of E^0, the better the reducing ability of the ions or compound, on moving downward.
3. Under standard conditions, any substance in this table will spontaneously oxidise any other substance lower to it.

8.3.1 Predicting the Cell EMF

e.g.: Let us consider the cell reaction

$$Zn(s)\ |Zn^{+2}\ (aq)\ ||\ Ag^+\ (aq)\ |\ Ag$$

By using the electro chemical series, predict the EMF of the cell

Solution: The EMF of the cell reaction can be calculated by using the formula

$$E^0_{cell} = E^0_{right} - E^0_{left}$$

$$= \text{Cathode potential} - \text{Anode potential}$$

$$= 0.80 - (-0.763)$$

$$= 0.80 + 0.763$$

$$= 1.563 \text{ v}$$

8.3.2 Predicting the Feasibility of the Reaction

The feasibility of a redox reaction can be easily predicted by using electro chemical series. The E^0_{cell} is calculated by using the formula.

$$E^0_{cell} = E^0_{cathode} - E_{anode}$$

If E^0_{cell} = +ve, the reaction is feasible

E^0_{cell} = –ve, the reaction is not feasible

e.g.: Consider the reaction

$$2Ag\,(s) + Zn^{+2}\,(aq) \rightarrow 2Ag^+\,(aq) + Zn(s) \text{ is feasible or not}$$

Solution: The Half-reactions are:

Anode: $2Ag\,(s) \rightarrow 2\,Ag^+\,(aq) + 2e^-$ $E^0 = 0.80$ V   .....(8.23)

Cathode: $Zn^{2+}(aq) + 2e^- \rightarrow Zn\,(s)$ $E^0 = -0.763$ V   .....(8.24)

$$E^0\,cell = E_{cathode} - E_{anode}$$

$$= -\,0.763 - 0.80$$

$$= -\,1.563$$

The reaction is not feasible

8.3.3 The Nernst Equation

Any half-cell reaction is written as a reaction i.e., acceptance of electron by the reactants to form the products.

$$\alpha(ox) + ne^- \quad\rightleftharpoons\quad \beta\,(Rd) \qquad .....(8.25)$$

(Reactants)   (products)

in which 'α' moles of oxidised species (ox) in the half-cell is reduced by a reaction involving n e$^-$ to 'β' moles of reduced species (Rd) in the half-cell. The change in the free energy for half-cell reduction is expressed according to the equation.

$$\Delta G = \Delta G^\circ + RT \ln \frac{\alpha\,(Rd)^\beta}{\alpha\,(ox)\alpha} \qquad .....(8.26)$$

where $\alpha(Rd)$ = arbitrary activity of the products,

$\alpha(ox)$ = arbitrary activity of the reactants

According to law of mass action, we raise the power which is equal to the number of moles of β of products or α of reactants.

Substituting –nFE and –nFE^0 into the equation (8.26) in the place of ΔG and ΔG°, we obtain,

$$-nFE = -nFE^0 + RT \, ln \, \frac{\alpha(Rd)^\beta}{\alpha(ox)^\alpha} \qquad \ldots(8.27)$$

$$E = E^0 - \frac{RT}{nF} \, ln \, \frac{\alpha \, (Rd)^\beta}{\alpha \, (ox)^\alpha} \qquad \ldots(8.28)$$

This equation is known as Nernst equation and in which E$^\circ$ is the standard potential i.e., when the activities of all the reactants and products are unity.

This equation is used to obtain individual electrode potential or cell emf from a known E^0 at a specific temperature, T, for a reaction involving n e$^-$ at specified activities of the reactants and products.

At standard temperature and pressure, the equation becomes

$$E = E^0 - \frac{0.0592}{n} \, log \, \frac{\alpha \, products}{\alpha \, reactants} \qquad \ldots(8.29)$$

The above equation is obtained by using this equation

$$E = E^0 - \frac{2.303RT}{nF} \, log \, k \qquad \ldots(8.30)$$

where   E^0 – Standard electrode potential

R – Gas constant

T = Kelvin temperature

n = No. of electrons transferred in the half reaction

F = Farady of electricity

K = equilibrium constant for half cell reaction as in equilibrium law.

When we are substituted with standard conditions the equation is obtained.

e.g.: Calculate the emf of the cell

$$Zn \mid zn^{+2} \, (0.001M) \parallel Ag^+ \, (0.1M) \mid Ag$$

Solution: The Half-cell reaction that occurred at anode and cathode are:

Cathode: $2 \, Ag^+ + 2e^- \rightarrow 2Ag \qquad E^0 = +0.80$

$$\text{Anode:} \quad Zn \quad \rightarrow \quad Zn^{2+} + 2e^- \qquad E^\circ = -0.76 \text{ v}$$

$$\text{Cell} = Zn + 2Ag+ \quad \rightleftharpoons \quad Zn^{2+} + 2Ag \quad E^0 = 1.56 \text{ v}$$

$$E_{cell} = E^0_{cell} - \frac{0.0591}{n} \log \frac{\alpha \text{ products}}{\alpha \text{ reactants}}$$

$$= 1.56 - \frac{0.059}{n} \log [zn^{+2}]/[Ag^{+2}]$$

$$= 1.56 - \frac{0.0591}{2} \log \frac{\left[10^{-3}\right]}{\left[10^{-1}\right]^2}$$

$$= 1.56 - 0.02955 \,(\log 10^{-1})$$

$$= 1.56 + 0.02955$$

$$= 1.58955 \text{ v}$$

What is the reduction potential at 25 °C of Pt wire electrodes immersed in acidic solution of ferrous ion at a concentration of 0.50 molal (m) and ferric ions at a concentration of 0.25 m. The activity coefficient α of the ferrous ion is 0.435 and for ferric ion is 0.390.

Solution: The cell reaction is represented as

$$Fe^{3+} + e^- \quad \rightleftharpoons \quad Fe^{2+}$$

The activity of each electrode is $\alpha = 0.435 \times 0.50 = 0.218$ for the ferrous ion and for the Ferric ion is $\alpha = 0.390 \times 0.25 = 0.0975$

$$E_{electrode} = E^0_{Fe3+ \rightarrow Fe2+} - \frac{0.0591}{1} \log \frac{\alpha Fe^{2+}}{Fe^{3+}}$$

$$= 0.771 - 0.0592 \log \frac{0.218}{0.0975}$$

$$= 0.771 - 0.021$$

$$E_{electrode} = 0.750 \text{ v}$$

8.4 Calculations

8.4.1 Calculation of Half Cell Potential

For an oxidation Half-cell reaction, when the metal electrode M gives M^{n+} ion.

$$M \rightarrow Mn^+ + ne^-$$

The Nernst equation takes the form

$$E = E^0 - \frac{2.303RT}{nF} \log \frac{\left[M^{n+}\right]}{\left[M\right]} \qquad \ldots\ldots(8.31)$$

When the concentration of solid metal $[M] = 0$, the nernst equation is written as

$$E = E^0 - \frac{2.303RT}{nF} \log [M^{n+}] \qquad \ldots\ldots(8.32)$$

Substituting the values of R, F, and T at 25 °C, the quantity $\dfrac{2.303\,RT}{F}$ becomes 0.0591. The nernst equation can be written in its simplified form as

$$E = E^0 - \frac{0.0591}{n} \log [\,M^{n+}] \qquad \ldots\ldots (8.33)$$

This is the equation for the oxidation Half-cell and in the case of reduction Half-cell, the sign will be reversed.

e.g.: what is the potential of a Half-cell consisting of zinc electrode in 0.01M $ZnSO_4$ solution at 25 °C, $E^0 = 0.763$ v

Solution : The Half-cell reaction is

$$Zn \rightarrow Zn^{2+} + 2e^-$$

The Nernst equation for the oxidation Half-cell reaction is

$$E = E^0 - \frac{0.0591}{n} \log [zn^{+2}]$$

where $\quad n = 2; \; E^0 = 0.763$ v

Substituting in the above equation

$$E = 0.763 - \frac{0.0591}{2} \log (0.01)$$

$$= 0.763 - \frac{0.0591}{2} \log 10^{-2}$$

$$= 0.763 - \frac{0.0591}{2} (-2) \times 1$$

$$= 0.763 + 0.0591 = 0.8221 \text{ v}$$

8.4.2 Calculation of Equilibrium Constant for the Cell Reaction

The Nernst equation for a cell is

$$E_{cell} = E^0_{cell} - \frac{0.0591}{n} \log k \qquad \qquad \dots (8.33)$$

at equilibrium. The cell reaction is balanced and the cell potential is zero.

Then, the equation becomes

$$0 = E^0_{cell} - \frac{0.0591}{n} \log k \qquad \qquad \dots (8.34)$$

$$\log k = \frac{nE^0_{cell}}{0.0591} \qquad \qquad \dots (8.35)$$

e.g: Calculate the equilibrium constant for the reaction between silver nitrate and metallic zinc.

Solution: The cell reaction is

$$2\,Ag^+ + Zn \rightleftharpoons Zn^{2+} + 2Ag \qquad \qquad E^0_{cell} = 1.56 \text{ v}$$

$$\log K = \frac{nE^0_{cell}}{0.0591}$$

$$0 = 1.56 - 0.03 \log k$$

$$-1.56 = -0.03 \log k$$

$$\log k = \frac{-1.56}{-0.03} = 52$$

$$K = 1 \times 10^{52}$$

8.4.3 Standard Electromotive Force of Cells

Consider a cell which consists of a hydrogen gas electrode as anode and silver-silver chloride electrode as the cathode immersed in an acquacious solution of hydrochloric acid.

$$Pt \mid H_2 \text{ (Patm)} \mid HCl \text{ (c, moles/litre) } AgCl \mid Ag$$

The overall cell reaction is determined by combining the 2 half-reaction at each electrode:

$$\frac{1}{2}\,H_2 = H^+ + e^- \qquad \qquad \dots (8.36)$$

$$Ag\,Cl + e^- = Ag + Cl^- \qquad \qquad \dots (8.37)$$

$$AgCl + \tfrac{1}{2} H_2 = H^+ + Ag + Cl^- \quad\quad\quad .....(8.38)$$

At 25°C, the emf of the cell is given by:

$$E = E^0 - \frac{0.0592}{1} \log \frac{\alpha H^+ \alpha Ag \alpha Cl^-}{\alpha AgCl\ \alpha H_2^{1/2}} \quad\quad .....(8.39)$$

The solid phases are assigned to 1 and the pressure of the hydrogen gas can be adjusted to 1 atm which behaves ideally and has an activity of 1, the equation becomes

$$E = E^0 - 0.0592 \log \alpha_{H^+} \alpha_{Cl^-} \quad\quad .....(8.40)$$

The individual ionic activities are referred to as mean ionic activities

$$E = E^0 - 0.0592 \log \gamma_{\pm}^2\ c_{H+}\ c_{Cl^-} \quad\quad .....(8.41)$$

Where $\gamma_{\pm}^2$ mean ionic activity coefficient for a solution of hydrochloric acid whose ionic concentrations are C_{H+} and C_{Cl^-} respectively.

According to the overall reaction for the cell, the concentrations of H^+ and Cl^- must be equal, the equation is expressed as

$$E = E^0 - 0.0592 \log \gamma_{\pm}^2\ c^2 \quad\quad .....(8.42)$$

where 'c' is the molar concentration of HCl in the solution. Equation can be rearranged as

$$E + 0.0592 \log c^2 = E^0 - 0.0592 \log \gamma_{\pm}^2 \quad\quad ..... (8.43)$$

(or)

$$E + 0.1184 \log c = E^0 - 0.1184 \log \gamma \pm \quad\quad ..... (8.44)$$

By using Debye-Huckel theory $\log r_{\pm}$ is replaced by $-AZ^2 \sqrt{\mu}$

where 'A' is a constant for a particular medium

$$Z = \text{valence of the ions}$$

$$\mu = \text{Ionic strength of the solution}$$

$$E + 0.1184 \log c = E^0 + 0.1184\ (0.509) \sqrt{\mu} \quad\quad .....(8.45)$$

(or)

$$E + 0.1184 \log c = E^0 + 0.0603 \sqrt{\mu} \quad\quad ..... (8.46)$$

Because
$$\mu = \frac{1}{2} \sum c_i z_1^2 \qquad\qquad ..... (8.47)$$

where $\qquad\qquad$ i = ionic species

then for the cell with only HCl in solution

$$E + 0.1184 \log c = E^0 + 0.0603 \sqrt{c} \qquad .....(8.48)$$

Debye-Huckel theory is applicable to dilute solutions. When we plot a graph between $\sqrt{c}$ and E^0 and extrapolating the line it intersects the vertical axis, yields a value of E^0 which corresponds to the EMF of the cell at infinite dilution.

e.g.: What is the standard potential E^0, for a cell consisting of a hydrogen gas electrode (p = 1 atm) as the anode and a silver-silver bromide electrode as the cathode immersed in a solution of 0.0004M hydrobromic acid. The EMF of cell is determined as 0.4745 volts.

The E^0 is find out.

$$Pt \mid H_2 \text{ (1 atm)} \mid HBr \text{ (0.0004M)} \mid AgBr \mid Ag$$

The overall cell reaction is

$$AgBr + \frac{1}{2} H_2 = H^+ + Ag + Br^-$$

$$E + 0.1184 \log c = E^0 + 0.0603 \sqrt{c}$$

$\therefore \qquad$
$$E^0 = E + 0.1184 \log c - 0.0603 \sqrt{c}$$

$$E^0 = 0.4745 - 0.4023 - 0.0012$$

$$= 0.071 \text{ volts}$$

According to Gibbs-Stockholm agreement, the measured emf should be designated as a reduction potential i.e., the unknown electrode is the cathode in the cell, the relative ability of the electrode to accept electron is measured as a reference electrode. The cell can be written as

$$E_{cell} = E_{reference} + E_{unknown\ electrode} \qquad .....(8.49)$$

where the unknown electrode is the right electrode in the cell.

If the potentials are determined under standard conditions, i.e., 25 °C, 1 atm pressure and unit activity of all species, then for the reduction potential

$$E^0_{cell} = E^0_{reference} + E^0_{unknown\ electrode} \qquad .....(8.50)$$

If the electrodes are connected, the reference electrode became the cathode and the unknown electrode became the anode, an oxidation potential would be determined. Oxidation potentials are not normally used for comparing cell potentials.

Oxidation potentials differ from reduction potentials only by having the reverse sign.

e.g.: Standard reduction potential for the silver-silver chloride electrode is + 0.223 volts its oxidation potential is – 0.223 volts.

The absolute potential of a single electrode cannot be measured; the relative potential can be measured by combining the electrode with reference electrode to form a cell.

Consider a cell that consists of a reference Hydrogen electrode and a second electrode whose potential is being determined. Then, the cell is represented as

$$E^0_{cell} = E^0_{H_2(anode)} + E^0_{unknown\,electrode(cathode)} \qquad .....(8.51)$$

Under unit Hydrogen ion activity and also under standard conditions, the reference Hydrogen electrode, which is primary reference electrode, the potential is arbitrarily assigned a potential of 0.000 Volts.

$$E^0_{H_2} = 0 \qquad ....(8.52)$$

Therefore, the $E^0_{cell} = E^0_{unknown\,electrode\,(cathode)}$

In addition to the Hydrogen electrode, secondary reference electrodes are such as 0.1N calomel electrode, 1N calomel electrode, saturated calomel electrode and the silver-silver chloride electrode. These electrodes can be standardised by using primary reference electrode i.e., Hydrogen electrode.

They are often use for laboratory measurement because they do not require any adjustment before use.

While handling the Hydrogen gas electrode, Hydrogen gas pressure must be controlled which requires careful handling and frequent adjustment.

HCl solution acts as the electrolyte solution in the secondary reference electrode which also acts as a salt bridge in order to maintain the electrical contact between the electrode and the rest of the cell.

It minimizes the potential difference that occurs across the liquid boundary and also mixing to any significant extent with the external solution by introducing a porous ceramic plug. The potential difference at this boundary is known as liquid junction potential.

In the cells containing liquid junction potential, the E of the cell is

$$E_{cell} = E_{anode} + E_{junction} + E_{cathode} \qquad .....(8.53)$$

8.5 Types of Electrodes

8.5.1 Standard and Formal Reduction Potentials

The standard reduction potentials can be calculated by taking one electrode as the reference electrode and the other electrode whose EMF is being determined in an electro chemical cell.

Where as formal reduction potential of an electrode is obtained by using specified concentration of all species. i.e., equal concentration of both oxidised and the reduced species.

- It is an experimentally observed value.

- This potential is obtained by considering the liquid junction potential, ionic strength, complexation and other variations which effect the EMF the cell.

e.g.: The standard reduction potential of the calomel electrode of unit activity of all species is + 0.268 v but the formal reduction potential of 0.1N calomel electrode is + 0.334 volts and the 1N calomel electrode is + 0.280 v and the saturated calomel electrode is + 0.242 v.

In some cases, the absolute potential cannot be obtained because of the limited solubility of species at these cases only formal reduction potentials are obtained.

1. Calculate the E^0_{cell} for an electrochemical cell consisting of a zinc electrode and a copper electrode each immersed in a solution of its ions at an activity of 1.00.

Solution:

The cell is written as

$$Zn|\ Zn^{2+}\ (\alpha = I)\ ||\ Cu^{+2}\ (\alpha = 1)\ |\ cu$$

The cell reaction is written as

$$Zn + Cu^{2+} = Zn^{2+} + Cu$$

$$E^0 cell = E^0\ left\ +\ E^0\ right$$
$$\qquad\qquad (oxidation)\ (reducrion)$$

$$=\ E^0_{Zn^{2+} \rightarrow Zn}\ +\ E^0_{Cu^{2+} \rightarrow Cu}$$
$$\qquad (oxidation)\ (reduction)$$

$$=\ E^0_{Zn^2 \rightarrow Zn}\ +\ E^0_{Cu^{+2} \rightarrow Cu}$$

$$= + 0.763 + (+ 0.337) = 1.00\ v$$

The '+' sign for the $-$ 0.763 $\rightarrow$ this value is the standard reduction potential as the Zn is oxidised; the sign gets changed.

2. Will a silver electrode reduce a lead electrode at 25 $^{\circ}$C when both the half cells are at unit activity?

Solution:

The reduction reactions of lead and silver are as follows:

$$Ag^+ + e^- = Ag \qquad\qquad E^0 = + 0.799$$

$$\frac{1}{2}\,Pb^{2+} + e^- = \frac{1}{2}\,Pb \qquad E^0 = -0.126$$

The silver potential is more positive when compared to the lead therefore silver is more reduced easily than lead. This Ag electrode cannot reduce the pb electrode and if the cell is written mistaken by considering the Ag electrode as the anode an the pb electrode as cathode, the cell potential becomes negative. In order to obtain the cell is +ve provide the flow of electron in the external circuit from anode to the cathode.

Note: The cell emf must always be positive where as the potentials of the individual electrodes can be either + ve or −ve.

The cell reaction is written as :

$$Ag \,|\, Ag^+ \,(\alpha = 1) \,||\, Pb^{+2} \,(\alpha = 1) \,|\, Pb$$

The overall reaction as

$$Ag + \frac{1}{2}\,Pb^{2+} = Ag^+ + \frac{1}{2}\,Pb$$

$$E^0_{cell} = E^0_{Ag \to Ag^+} + E^0_{pb^{2+} \to pb} = -0.799 + (-0.126)$$

$$= -0.925 \text{ v}$$

This results in wrong potential because E^0 is − ve ; i.e., the mistake can be corrected by reversing the electrodes.

$$Pb \,|\, Pb^{2+} \,(\alpha = 1) \,||\, Ag^+ \,(\alpha = 1) \,|\, Ag$$

$$Ag^+ + \frac{1}{2}\,Pb = Ag + \frac{1}{2}\,Pb^{2+}$$

$$E^0_{cell} = E^0_{Pb \to Pb^{2+}} + E^0_{Ag^+ \to Ag}$$

$$= +0.126 + (+0.799)$$

$$= +0.925 \text{ v}$$

8.5.2 Configuration of a Cell

E.g: What is the configuration for a cell composed of a ferrocyanide-ferricyanide electrode and a mercurous-mercuric electrode when both half-cells are at unit activity at 25 °C? This type of cell is known as oxidation-reduction system.

Sol: $\quad Fe(CN)_6^{3-} + e^- \rightarrow Fe(CN)_6^{4-} \qquad E^0 = +0.356$

$$Hg^{+2} + e^- \rightarrow \frac{1}{2} Hg_2^{+2} \qquad E^0 = +0.907$$

The mercurous-mercuric electrode has a larger reduction potential and therefore will oxidize the ferrocyanide to ferricyanide. The cell is written as:

$$Pt \mid Fe(CN)_6^{3-}, Fe(CN)_6^{4-} \ (\alpha = 1) \parallel Hg^{+2}, Hg_2^{2+} \ (\alpha = 1) \mid pt$$

The over cell reaction is

$$Fe(CN)_6^{4-} + Hg^{2+} \quad = \quad Fe(CN)_6^{3-} + \frac{1}{2} Hg_2^{2+}$$

The calculated E^0_{cell} is

$$E^0_{cell} = E^0_{Fe(CN)_6^{4-}} \rightarrow Fe(CN)_6^{3-} + E^0_{Hg^{+2}} \rightarrow \frac{1}{2} Hg_2^{2+}$$

$$= -0.356 + (+0.907)$$

$$= 0.551 \text{ volts}$$

2. Calculate the emf of the following cell at 25 °C.

$$Ag, Ag\,I \mid I^- \ (\alpha = 0.4) \parallel Cl^- \ (\alpha = 0.8) \mid AgCl, Ag$$

Sol: The cell Reaction is

$$I^- + Agcl = AgI + Cl$$

$$\Rightarrow \quad n = 1 \text{ apply this in the nernst equation}$$

$$E_{cell} = E^0_{cell} - \frac{0.0592}{1} \log \frac{\alpha_{AgI} \ \alpha_{Cl^-}}{\alpha_I - \alpha_{AgCl}}$$

$$= E^0_{cell} = E^0_{I \rightarrow AgI} + E^0_{Agcl \rightarrow Cl^-} \qquad \text{i.e., activities of the solids} = 1$$

$$= +0.156 + (+0.223)$$

$$= +0.379 \text{ volts}$$

$$E_{cell} = 0.379 - 0.018 = +0.361 \text{ v}$$

Types of Electrodes

The different types of electrodes are:

(a)   Metal-Metal ion electrodes

(b)   Amalgam electrodes

(c)   Metal-Insoluble electrodes

(d)   Oxidation-Reduction electrode

(e)   Gas electrodes

(f)   Membrane electrode

(g)   Micro electrode

(a)   Metal-Metal ion Electrode: The Daniel cell consists of electrodes of this type. Each electrode is made simply by immersing a metal strip into a solution containing ions of the metal.

e.g: Nickel electrode

$$\text{Ni} \mid \text{Ni}^{+2} \text{ (c, moles/ liter)}$$

(b)   Amalgam Electrodes: In this the metal electrode is replaced by a metal amalgam immersed in a solution containing metal ion.

An advantage is that the active metals such as sodium or potassium react with amalgam an their salts.

e.g.: Sodium-Amalgam electrode

The cell is represented as,

$$\text{Na (in Hg at } c_1\text{, Moles/ liter)} \mid \text{Na}^+ \text{ (c, Moles/ liter)}$$

(c)   Metal-In Soluble Electrode:

The examples for this type of electrodes are calomel electrode (Mercurous chloride) and the silver-silver chloride electrode.

They are widely used as reference electrodes.

Reference electrodes produce an invariant potential that is not affected by changes in solution concentration.

They are used with another electrode called the indicator electrode which was in reversible cells.

Calomel Electrode: It consists of Mercury, a paste of mercurous chloride and a solution of KCl which provides chloride ions. The electrode is represented by:

$$\text{Hg} \mid \text{Hg}_2 \, Cl_2 \mid Cl^- \qquad \text{(c, moles/liter)}$$

The electrode Reaction is

$$Hg = Hg^+ + e^- \qquad\qquad .....(8.54)$$

$$Hg^+ + Cl^- = \frac{1}{2} Hg_2 Cl_2 \qquad\qquad .....(8.55)$$

$$--------------------------------$$

$$Hg + Cl^- = \frac{1}{2} Hg_2 Cl_2 + e^- \qquad\qquad ..... (8.56)$$

$$--------------------------------$$

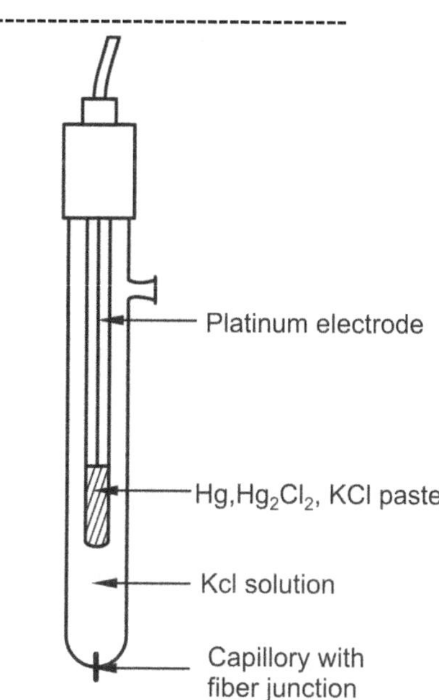

Fig. 8.3 Calomel electrode.

Silver-silver Chloride Electrode: It consists of a layer of silver chloride on a silver wire which was immersed in a solution containing chloride ions. The electrode is represented by,

$$Ag \,|\, AgCl \,|\, Cl^- \qquad (c, moles/|\ liter)$$

And the electrode reactions is

$$Ag = Ag^+ + e^- \qquad\qquad .....(8.57)$$

$$Ag^+ + Cl^- = AgCl \qquad\qquad .....(8.58)$$

$$-----------------------$$

$$Ag + Cl^- = AgCl + e^- \qquad\qquad .....(8.59)$$

$$-----------------------$$

(d) Oxidation-Reduction Electrode

Every electro chemical half-cell involves an oxidation reduction reaction. The Half-cells which posses inert electrode immersed in a solution containing both oxidized and Reduced forms of substance are called oxidation-reduction electrodes.

The electrode may either functions as cathode or anode.

The electrode reaction depends upon the potential of the electrode in a cell

Platinum (Pt) is the most widely used metal for inert electrodes

Gold and silver have limited usefulness as inert electrodes because both are soft and in addition, the silver prone to oxidation.

A platinum wire is immersed in a solution containing ferrous and ferric ions belongs to the categories of oxidation-reduction electrode.

The electrode is abbreviated as:

$$Pt \,|\, Fe^{+2} \,(c_1,\ moles/\ liter),\ Fe^{+3} \,(c_2,\ moles/\ liter)$$

The electrode reaction for that half-cell is :

$$Fe^{+2} = Fe^{+3} + e^- \qquad\qquad .....(8.60)$$

Oxidation-redction electrode may also be made with organic substances such as. Quinhydrone.

Quinhydrone is an equimolar mixture of Benzoquinone, (Q). Hydroquinone (H_2Q)

These substances are slightly soluble in water

It involves reversible oxidation-reduction reaction

OH — + 2H$_2$O $\rightleftharpoons$ O — + 2H$_3$O$^+$ + 2e$^-$ — OH — O

Hydroquinone, H$_2$O   Benzoquinone, Q

When a platinum wire is introduced into this, the oxidation-reduction electrode is produced. The electrode can be written as:

$$Pt \,|\, H_2Q,\ Q,\ H_3O^+ \ (c\ moles\,/\,liter)$$

The potential of the Quinhydrone electrode varies with the H_3O^+ concentration i.e. p^H can be maintained

(e) Gas Electrodes

The inert metal wire is bubbled over a gas and the metal wire is placed in a solution containing ions that can be derived from the gas produces gas electrode.

A platinum electrode which is coated with colloidal platinum black.

This was done in order to increase the effective surface area and facilitates the electrode reaction.

e.g: Hydrogen electrode

$$Pt \mid H_2 \text{ (known pressure)} \mid H^+ \text{ (c, moles / liter)}$$

and the electrode reaction is represented as:

$$Pt + H_2 = Pt\,H_2 \qquad\qquad .....(8.61)$$

$$Pt\,H_2 = Pt + \frac{1}{2}\,H^+ + e^- \qquad\qquad .....(8.62)$$

$$H_2 = \frac{1}{2}H^+ + e^- \qquad\qquad .....(8.63)$$

(f) Membrane Electrode

A thin, ion-sensitive glass membrane encloses an electrolyte solution. The electrodes are placed in the electrolyte solutions which detect potentials arising at the glass/ solution interface. By controlling the composition of the glass or crystalline membrane, the electrodes are particularly sensitive to certain ions in the solution. The p^H electrode is the most common type of membrane electrode. It consists of a platinum wire which was dipped into the solution of Hydrochloric acid. The Pt wire is in contact with the internal reference electrode. Internal reference electrode may be silver-silver chloride electrode, calomel electrode, which was sealed in a high resistance body. This electrode is responsive to protons and other monovalent ions but relatively unresponsive to divalent ions:

By carefully adjusting the three-dimensional arrangement of cations such as Na^+, Ca^{+2}, Li^+ and Ba^{+2} located in the silicate structure of glass membrane, one can control the responsiveness of the electrode to monovalent cations other than Hydrogen.

e.g: The glass p^H electrode produces a sodium error which shows responsiveness to sodium ions at high p^H values. This error can be minimized by employing high concentration of lithium ions incorporated in the silicate matrix

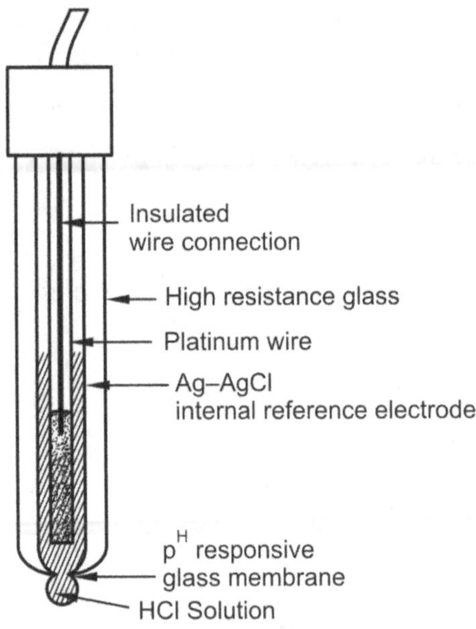

Fig. 8.4 Glass (Membrane) electrode.

The glass membrane p^H electrode is represented as:

Internal reference | Pt | HCl (c, moles/liter) | Glass membrane | External solution

Electrode

In order to obtain a complete cell, the external reference electrode is combined with glass electrode. If two glass electrodes are immersed in the same solution and connected to a p^H meter, a small potential difference can be noted between the electrodes. This is mainly due to the slight differences in the properties of the individual glass membrane and for the p^H measurement. This individual electrode variation requires standardization of each cell containing a glass electrode against a buffer of known p^H.

The thin membranes may also be fabricated from cellulose, polyethylene, Colloidon or liquid-ion-exchange resins that are insoluble in water. Salt-crystals can also be used in the place of glass as ion-selective membrane electrode.

(g) **Micro Electrodes**

These are very small enough to make a contact with a single cell or neutral unit in an intact animal.

They possess tapered needless which is made up of metal or glass.

- The diameter of the electrode is in the order of $1\,\mu$ or less
- The electrode is like that of a small hypodermic needle or pipette.
- This electrode is sterilized and implanted in an animal for pharmacological studies.

Types of Electrodes

For an electro chemical cell, two electrodes are required. Based upon the usage, they are classified into:

(a)   Reference electrode

(b)   Indicator electrode

Reference Electrodes: A reference electrode is one which produces a constant potential in which the potential is not affected by changes in the concentration of the solution.

The reference electrode is taken as cathode and the unknown electrode is considered as anode then the oxidation potential is obtained and the reduction potential is obtained by reversing the sign.

e.g.: The standard reduction potential of silver-silver chloride electrode is + 0.223 volts and its oxidation potential is – 0.223 v. Again, the reference electrodes are of two types. They are:

(a)   Primary reference electrode

   e.g.: Hydrogen electrode

(b)   Secondary reference electrode

   e.g.: Calomel electrode and silver-silver chloride electrode

   Secondary reference electrodes are often used and they do not require any adjustment. They are standardised by using 1^0 reference electrode.

   A KCl solution is used as a salt bridge. The functions of the salt bridge is discussed previously.

Hydrogen Gas Electrode

This was discussed under different type of electrodes.

Advantages:

It is a reversible electrode with respect to hydrogen ion

Used in the determination of pH of solution

Used as a primary reference standard

Disadvantages:

It is difficult to handle hydrogen electrode.

Calomel Electrode

Advantages

It is used as a reference electrode and indicator electrode.

Used in the determination of pH of a solution.

Silver-silver Chloride Electrode

Advantages

It is used as a reference electrode and is combined with an indicator electrode

Used in the determination of pH of a solution.

Reversible and stable electrode

Can be combined with the cells containing chlorides without inserting liquid junction.

Concentration Cells

In a concentration cell, the emf is produced due to the differences in the activities of solutions of the same materials constituting the two cells.

Concentration cell is a galvanic cell in which electrical energy is produced by the transfer of material from a system of high concentration to low concentration.

These all of two types:

    (a)   Electrode concentration cells

    (b)   Electrolyte concentration cells

Applications

- Useful in the estimation of solubility of sparingly soluble salts.
- Useful in the evaluation of valence of an ion.
- Useful in the determination of transition point.

Electrode Concentration Cells

In an electrode concentration cell, emf is produced when two electrodes of different concentrations are dipped in the same concentration of solution of the same electrolyte.

Two hydrogen electrodes at unequal gas pressures p_1 and p_2 are immersed in the solution of hydrogen ions. The cell is represented as:

$$Pt, H_2 \ (pH_2 = p_1) \mid H^+ \mid H_2 \ (pH_2 = p_2), Pt$$

If $p_1 > p_2$, oxidation of hydrogen gas takes place at the left hand electrode and reduction of hydrogen ions takes place at the right-hand electrode.

The EMF is independent of concentration of hydrogen ions in which the electrodes are immersed.

The EMF is expressed as:

$$E = \frac{RT}{2F} ln \frac{p_1}{p_2} \qquad \text{.....(8.64)}$$

In the amalgam cells, the concentration of electrodes are expressed the emf of the cell is expressed as:

$$E = \frac{RT}{2F} ln \frac{c_1}{c_2} \qquad \text{.....(8.65)}$$

Electrolyte Concentration Cells

In electrolyte concentration cells, the electrodes are identical but the electrolyte solutions have different concentrations.

The difference in the concentration produces a change in potential. The source of electrical energy is the tendency of the electrolyte to diffuse from a solution of higher concentration to lower concentration. After a lapse of time, the two concentrations of the electrolyte are equal. The emf of the concentration cell is maximum at the start and gradually falls to zero as the two concentrations become identical.

e.g.: An electrochemical cell with zinc electrodes and the solution of zinc sulphate of two different concentrations c_1 and c_2 joining together through a salt bridge.

The cell system is represented as

$$Zn \mid Zn^{2+} (c_{1)} \parallel Zn^{2+} (c_2) \mid Z_n$$

The emf of the cell is expressed as:

$$E = \frac{RT}{2F} ln \frac{c_1}{c_2}$$

Suppose a cell consists of 2 copper electrodes immersed in $CuSO_4$ solution at 25 °C having activities of 0.01 and 0.05 respectively.

The cell is represented by

$$Cu \mid Cu^{2+} (\alpha_1 = 0.01) \parallel Cu^{2+} (\alpha_2 = 0.05) \mid Cu$$

The reactions at the anode and the cathode are

At anode $\qquad Cu = Cu^{+2} (\alpha_1 = 0.01) + 2e^-$

At cathode $\qquad Cu^{2+} (\alpha_2 = 0.05) + 2e^- = Cu$

The overall reaction is

$$Cu^{+2} (\alpha_2 = 0.05) = Cu^{+2} (\alpha_1 = 0.01)$$

The corresponding Nernst equation for individual electrodes are

$$E_{left} = E^0_{\underset{(oxn)}{Cu \to Cu^{2+}}} - \frac{0.0592}{2} \log \alpha_1 \qquad \dots(8.66)$$

$$E_{rright} = E^0_{\underset{(oxn)}{Cu^{2+} \to Cu}} - \frac{0.0592}{2} \log \alpha_2 \qquad \dots(8.67)$$

The equation for the cell emf is

$$E_{cell} = E_{left} + E_{right} \qquad \dots(8.68)$$

$$= \left(E^0_{Cu \to Cu^{+2}} - \frac{0.0592}{2} \log \alpha_1 \right) + \left(E^0_{Cu^{+2} \to Cu} - \frac{0.0592}{2} \log \frac{1}{\alpha_2} \right)$$

$$= \left(E^0_{Cu \to Cu^{+2}} + E^0_{Cu^{+2} \to Cu} \right) - \frac{0.0592}{2} \log \frac{\alpha_1}{\alpha_2} \qquad \dots(8.69)$$

From this the general equation becomes

$$E_{cell} = \frac{0.0592}{n} \log \frac{\alpha_1}{\alpha_2} \qquad \dots(8.70)$$

The electrolyte at the higher activity α_2, bends to diffuse spontaneously into the solution of lower activity and the emf of the cell rises due to difference in effective concentrations.

Problems

1. Calculate the EMF of a cell whose $E^0_{cu \to cu^{2+}} = -0.337$ and $E^0 cu^{2+} \to +\omega = +0.337$ and their activities are 0.01 and 0.05 respectively.

Sol: The equation is represented as:

$$E_{cell} = -\frac{0.0592}{2} \log \frac{0.01}{0.05} \quad = 0.021 \text{ v}$$

2. Calculate the EMF at 25 °C arising from the cell

$$Ag; Ag\,Cl \mid Cl^- \,(\alpha_2 : 0.10 \parallel Cl^- \,(\alpha_1 = 0.01) \mid Hg_2Cl_2, Hg$$

Sol: The overall reaction is :

$$Ag + Cl^- \,(\alpha_2 = 0.10) + \frac{1}{2} Hg_2\,Cl_2 = AgCl + Hg + Cl^- \,(\alpha_1 = 0.01)$$

The Nernst equation for individual electrodes

$$E_{right} = E^0_{Cl^- \to AgCl} - \frac{0.0592}{1} \log \frac{\alpha AgCl}{\alpha Ag \alpha Cl^-}$$

(oxidation)

$$E_{right} = E^0_{\frac{1}{2}Hg_2Cl_2 \to Cl^-} - \frac{0.0592}{1} \log \frac{\alpha Hg \alpha Cl^-}{\alpha Hg_2Cl_2}$$

(reduction)

The equation for the cell EMF is

$$E_{cell} = E_{left} + E_{right}$$

The activity of all the solids is unity and the cell EMF becomes

$$E_{cell} = E^0_{Cl^- \to AgCl} - 0.0592 \log \frac{1}{\alpha_2} + E^0_{\frac{1}{2}Hg_2Cl_2 \to cl^-} - 0.0592 \log \alpha_1$$

$$E_{cell} = (-0.223 - 0.0592 \log \frac{1}{0.10}) + (+0.268 - 0.0592 \log 0.01)$$

$$= -0.282 + 0.386 = +0.104 \text{ v}$$

Electrometric Determination of pH

The calomel electrode and silver chloride electrode are more convenient as reference electrodes and used commercially as pH meters.

The National Bureau of standards (NBS) determines the pH of its standard buffer. They determine the p^H by employing Hydrogen-indicating electrode and silver-silver chloride reference electrode

The electrodes which are used in the determination of pH are :

1. Hydrogen electrode,

2. Quinhydrone electrode,

3. Glass electrode.

1. *Hydrogen electrode*: A Standard Hydrogen electrode is coupled with another calomel electrode which contains the solution of unknown p^H. In both half-cells, hydrogen gas is used at 1 atm pressure at 25°C. The EMF of the cell is

$$Pt\ H_2\ (1\ atm)\ |\ H_3\ O^+\ (\alpha H^+ = ?)\ ||\ Cl\ (sat),\ Hg_2Cl_2\ |\ Hg$$

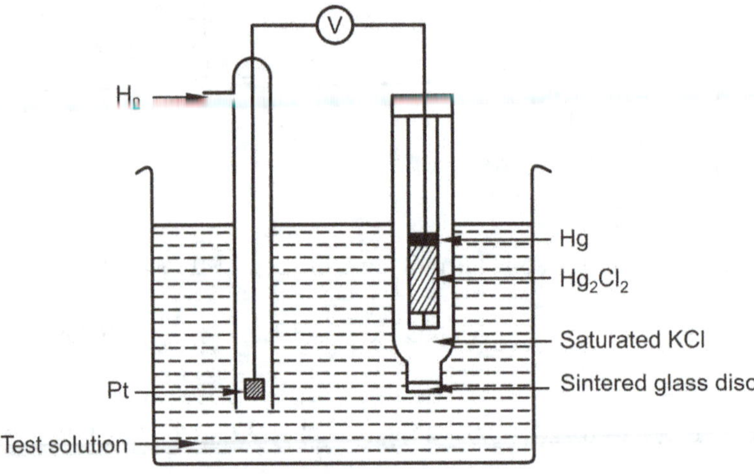

Fig. 8.5 A calomel electrode is coupled with unknown hydrogen electrode in the electrometric determination of pH by employing hydrogen electrode.

The Half-cell reactions are as follows:

At anode: left (oxidation) :

$$H_2 + 2H_2O = 2H_3O^+ (\alpha\ H^+ = ?) + 2e^- \qquad\qquad .....(8.71)$$

At cathode: Right (Reduction)

$$Hg_2Cl_2 + 2e^- = 2Cl^- + 2Hg \qquad\qquad .....(8.72)$$

Overall Reaction:

$$H_2 + Hg_2\ Cl_2 + 2H_2O = 2H_3O^+ + 2Hg + 2\ Cl^- \qquad\qquad .....(8.73)$$

where αH^+ represents the hydrogen ion activity of the test solution

The EMF of the cell is given by

$$E_{cell} = E_{H_2 \rightarrow 2H_3O^+} + E_{Hg_2Cl_2 \rightarrow Hg} \qquad\qquad ..... (8.74)$$

The potential of the Hydrogen electrode at 25°C and at a partial pressure of the Hydrogen gas at 1 atm is written as

$$E_{H_2} = E^0_{H_2 \rightarrow H_3O^+} - 0.0592 \log \frac{\alpha_{H_3O^+}}{1\ atm} \qquad\qquad ..... (8.75)$$

Under these conditions $E^0 = 0$ and the equation becomes

$$E_{H_2} = -0.0592 \log \alpha_{H_3O^+} \qquad\qquad .....(8.76)$$

and because $\quad pH = -\log \alpha_{H_3O^+}$

$$E_{H2} = 0.0592\ pH \qquad\qquad .....(8.77)$$

e.g: The potential of the saturated KCl calomel electrode in the reduction reaction is + 0.242 volts at 25^0C. Calculate the E cell.

Sol :
$$E_{cell} = 0.0592\ pH + 0.242 \qquad\qquad ..... (8.78)$$

$$pH = \frac{E_{cell} - 0.242}{0.0592} \qquad\qquad ..... (8.79)$$

E.g: A solution is placed between the Hydrogen electrode and the calomel electrode. The EMF of the cell is + 0.963 v at 25 ^{0}C. What is the p^H of the solution?

Sol:
$$pH = \frac{0.963 - 0.242}{0.0592}$$

$$= 12.2$$

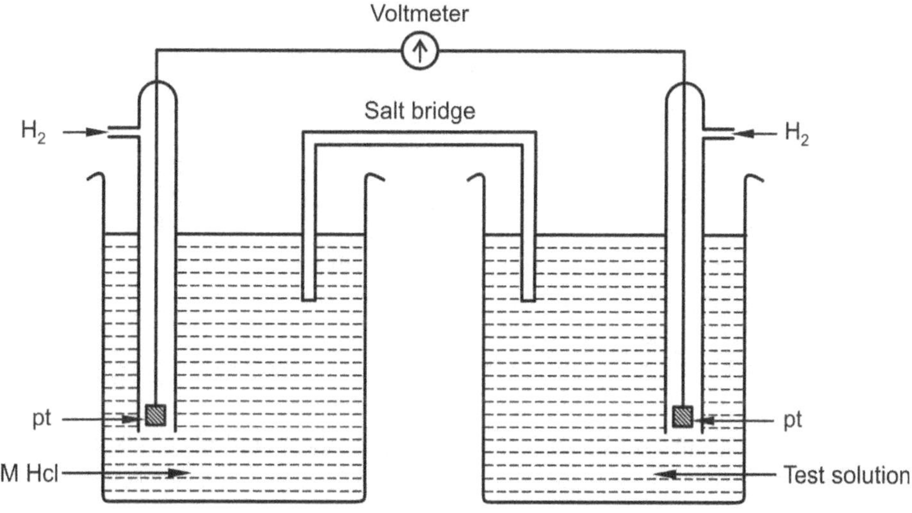

Fig. 8.6 Determination of pH with hydrogen electrode.

If another Hydrogen electrode is placed instead of calomel electrode and maintaining the Hydrogen gas in both half-cells at 1 atm pressure at 25 ^{0}C

The cell is represented as

$$Pt \mid H_2 \text{ (1 atm)} \mid H^+ \text{ (1M)} \mid\mid H^+ \text{ (unknown)} \mid H_2 \text{ (1 atm)} \mid Pt$$

The second electrode reaction is

$$H^+ + e^- \rightleftharpoons \frac{1}{2} H_2$$

The electrode potential of the second Half-cell is given by Nernst equation:

$$E = E^0 + \frac{2.303RT}{nF} \log \frac{\left[H^+ \right]}{pH_2^{1/2}} \qquad \qquad \dots\dots (8.80)$$

Since $pH_2^{1/2} = 1$ and $E^0 = 0$, we have

$$E = \frac{2.303RT}{nF} \log [H^+] \qquad \qquad \dots\dots (8.81)$$

Substituting the Value of R, T, n and F, the expression becomes

$$E = 0.0591 \log (H^+] \qquad \qquad \dots\dots (8.82)$$

$$E = -0.0591\ pH \qquad \qquad \dots\dots (8.83)$$

or

The emf of the cell, E_{cell} is given by:

$$E_{cell} = E_{right} - E_{left}$$

$$E_{left} = 0 \text{ (standard Hydrogen electrode is E = 0)}$$

$$E_{cell} = E_{right} = -(-0.05921)\ pH \qquad \qquad \dots\dots (8.84)$$

$$E_{right} = -(-0.0591 \times pH) = 0.0591 \times pH \qquad \qquad \dots\dots (8.85)$$

$$pH = \frac{E_{cell}}{0.059} \qquad \qquad \dots (8.86)$$

Merits:

It gives the absolute values of p^H while the other electrodes yield relative values.

Demerits:

It is not convenient for routine measurement

The Hydrogen gas is difficult to setup and transport.

Requires considerable volume of test solutions.

The test solution might poison the surface of Platinum etc., electrode.

The potential of electrode is altered by changes in barometric pressure.

e.g: The EMF of the following cell at 25 ^{0}C is 0.445v

$$Pt, H_2 \,(1 \text{ atm}) \,|\, H^+ \,(\text{test solution}) \,|\, KCl \text{ saturated solution} \,|\, Hg_2Cl_2 \,|\, Hg$$

Sol: $E_{cell} = 0.445$ v (given)

$$= 0.2415 - 0 = 0.2415 \text{ v}$$

Using the reaction

$$E_{cell} = E_{right} - E_{left}$$

$$0.445 = 0.2415 - (-0.0591 \times pH)$$

$$\Rightarrow \quad 0.445 = 0.2415 + 0.0591 \times pH$$

$$pH = \frac{0.445 - 0.2415}{0.0591}$$

$$= \frac{0.235}{0.0591}$$

$$= 3.44$$

Glass Electrode: The glass membrane electrode is typical of the membrane types electrodes.

It is most widely used pH-indicating electrode. The conventional electrode includes an acidic electrolyte solution of 0.1N HCl and internal silver-silver chloride reference electrode.

It is coupled with standard calomel electrode.

The EMF of the complete cell

$$Ag, Ag\,Cl \,|\, 1M\,HCl \,|\, Glass \,|\, \text{solution of unknown pH} \,\|\, KCl \,(sat) \,Hg_2\,Cl_2 \,|\, Hg$$

$$(\alpha_{H3O+} = ?)$$

The pH of the unknown solution is obtained from the cell EMF if the pH of the internal solution, 0.1N HCl is constant.

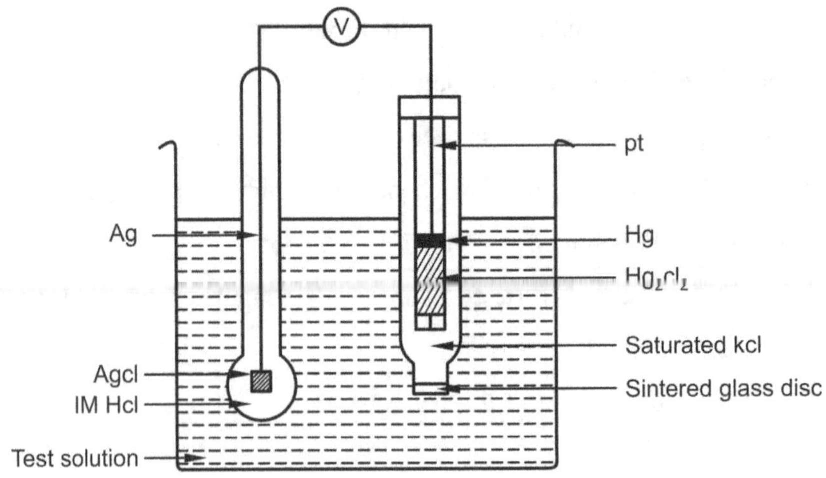

Fig. 8.6 Determination of pH using glass electrode.

The EMF of the cell at 25 ^{0}C results from the four separate potentials arising at separate interface

$$E_{cell} = E_{SCE} + E_{Asym} - E_{AgCl, Ag} + 0.059 \ (pH_{unknwon} - pH_{HCl\ solution}) \qquad ....(8.87)$$

where

E_{SCE} = Electromotive force of the standard calomel electrode

E_{Asym} = Electromotive force of the asymmetric electrode.

E_{SCE} arises at the boundary of Hg_2Cl_2 | Hg where as E_{Asy} arises at from the two boundaries of the glass membrane which is equivalent to difference in resistance that is arise owing to the manufacture.

$E_{AgCl,Ag}$ arises at the boundary Ag | AgCl.

pH_{HCl} solution is the p^H of the 0.1N HCl solution and pH unknown is the pH of the solution which is to be determined.

The asymmetrical potential may be associated with mechanical properties of the glass membrane, which effect the unequal mobility or absorption of ions on the two sides of the membrane.

E_{Asym} potential varies from one glass membrane to another by considering one glass electrode the E_{Asym} can be considered as constant.

The equation can be simplified at 25 °C to give

$$E_{cell} = E_{constant} + 0.0592 \, p^H{}_{unknown} \qquad \qquad \ldots\ldots (8.88)$$

$$pH = \frac{E_{cell} - E_{constant}}{0.0592} \qquad \qquad \ldots\ldots (8.89)$$

where $E_{constant}$ is the sum of all the boundary potentials in the cell plus constant potential arising from the 0.1N HCl solution.

The value of $E_{constant}$ cannot be determined accurately because of the variation in E_{Asym} from one glass electrode to another. This is not necessary as the pH meter can be standardised using a reference buffer.

The pH of a reference buffer measured with glass electrode is

$$pH_s = \frac{E_s - E_{constant}}{0.0592} \qquad \qquad \ldots\ldots (8.90)$$

where pH_s is the pH

         E_s = Emf of the National Bureau reference buffer solution.

Subtracting from to eliminate $E_{constant}$ the expression becomes

$$pH - pH_s = \frac{E_{cell} - E_s}{0.0592} \qquad \qquad \ldots\ldots (8.91)$$

$$pH = pH_s + \frac{E_{cell} - E_s}{0.0592} \qquad \qquad \ldots\ldots (8.92)$$

In the actual measurement of pH, a standardization dial is present on the pH meter. The pH meter is adjusted manually until the needle on the scale reads the pH of a reference buffer solution.

- For accurate determination, it is buffers to use two reference buffers. The buffers should be selected in such a way that one with a pH below and the other with a pH above that for unknown solution.

- The pH meter is similar in operation with potentiometer except its function with a high input resistance associated with the glass electrode.

- The chemical composition of the glass membrane is response to the pH of the solution.

- At high pH values a negative deviation is occurred. The theoretical potential is found with glass membranes containing high proportion of sodium ions.

- The sodium error may be arised due to high pH values

In strongly acidic solutions, a positive deviation from the theoretical EMF may be occurred. This error is believed due to decrease in the activity of rate, which may be in the ability of the solution to hydrate the membrane surface and the ions in solutions. Electrodes reduce the sodium error by incorporating a high proportion of lithium ions into the glass lattice.

It is not affected by oxidation-reduction systems but can be affected by cation exchange between the glass and the solution.

- The lithium ions incorporated in the glass do not exchange with other cations in the glass, unlike the sodium ions. This decrease in the ion exchange property produces a more stable glass lattice with a decrease sodium ion exchange at high pH values i.e. a reduction in alkaline error.

- A modern innovation in pH electrode is the combination electrode. In this a standard calomel electrode is in combination with reference electrode junction. Both the electrodes are embedded within a single body.

- It is a complex electrode system and they can detect the change in the pH with small samples.

- Another development is the use of fiber-optics sensor which allows the measurement of pH within a single living cell.

Merits:

It is Universally used because:

(a) It is simple to operate,

(b) It is not easily poisoned

(c) Its activity is not affected by strong oxidizing and reducing agents.

Demerits:

E^0_{cell} depends upon a particular glass electrode and hence it is not a universal constant and it also changes with time. Hence a glass electrode only compares pH values while the Hydrogen electrode measures pH absolutely.

Measurement of pH by using Quinhydrone Electrode

A platinum electrode is suspended in a solution whose pH is to be determined. The solution is saturated with Quimhydrone compound. This Half-cell is then combined with a standard calomel electrode (SCE). The complete cell can be represented as

SCE || solution of unknown pH saturated with quinhydrone || Pt

The EMF of the complete cell [E_{cell}] is determined with the help of a voltmeter.

The reduction half-cell reaction of quinhydrone electrode is

$$Q + 2H^+ + 2e^- \;\rightleftharpoons\; QH_2 \qquad \qquad \text{..... (8.93)}$$

The potential, E_Q of the quinhydrone electrode depends on the concentration of H^+ ions in solution.

From the Nernst equation:

$$E_Q = E_Q^0 - \frac{2.303RT}{F} \log \left[H^+ \right] \qquad \qquad \text{..... (8.94)}$$

$$E_Q = E_Q^0 + \frac{2.303RT}{F} \, pH \qquad \qquad \text{..... (8.95)}$$

The standard Reduction potential E_Q^0 of the quinhydrone electrode is 0.6996

Therefore $E_Q = 0.6996 = 0.591 \, pH$ $\qquad \qquad$ ..... (8.96)

We know that

$$E_{cell} = E_{right} - E_{left}$$

$$E_{cell} = E_Q - E_{SCE} \qquad \qquad \text{..... (8.97)}$$

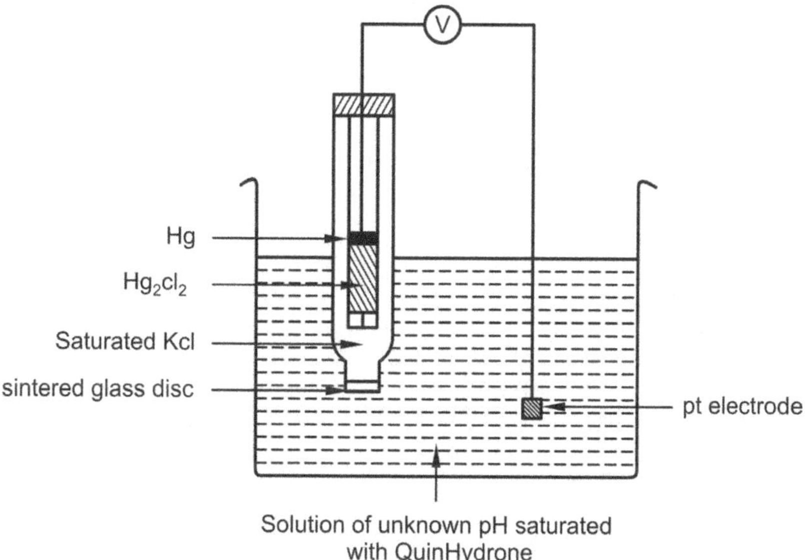

Fig. 8.7 Determination of pH using quinhydrone electrode.

The EMF of the standard calomel electrode is 0.2415

The value of E_Q from eq. 8.95, we have

$$E_{cell} = 0.6996 + 0.0591 \times pH - 0.2415 \qquad \qquad \text{..... (8.98)}$$

$$0.0591\ pH = 0.4581 - E_{cell} \qquad \qquad \text{..... (8.99)}$$

$$pH = \frac{0.4581 - E_{cell}}{0.0591} \qquad \qquad \text{..... (8.100)}$$

Merits

- It is easy to set up by immersing a platinum wire strip in test solution.
- The values of pH are very accurate in the presence of oxidizing ions which interfere with the working of a Hydrogen electrode.

Demerits

It does not give satisfactory result for solutions whose pH is more than 8.5 due to ionization or oxidation of hydroquinone.

Example: Find the pH of a solution placed in a hydroquinone half cell which was coupled with standard calomel electrode. The EMF of the combined cell was determined to be 0.123 v at 25°C.

$$E_{calomel} = 0.2415\ v \qquad \qquad E_Q^0 = 0.6996\ v$$

Solution: $\qquad E_{cell} = E_Q - E_{SCA}$

We know that

$$E_Q = E_Q^0 - \frac{2.303RT}{F}\ pH$$

$$= 0.6996 - 0.0591\ pH$$

Substituting $\quad EQ\ \&\ E_{SCA}$ in the above equation

$$0.123 = (0.6996 - 0.0591\ pH) - 0.2415$$

$$= 0.4581 - 0.0591\ pH$$

$$pH = \frac{0.4581 - 0.123}{0.0591}$$

$$pH = \frac{0.3351}{0.0591} = 5.67$$

A Summary of pH Definitions

1. It was first introduced by Sorensen and he gave the definition of pH as
$pH = - \log [H_3O^+]$

2. The concentration of Hydronium ion is replaced by the activity and the definition becomes

$$pH = - \log \alpha \, [H_3O^+] \qquad \qquad ....(8.101)$$

3. It is not possible by experimental means to measure the activity of single ion. The pH that is given by involving the activity is closely related to thermodynamic definition.

$$pH = - \log \alpha \, [H_3O^+]$$

This equation is known as the operational or experimental pH, does not correspond exactly to the pH on the activity scale because the junction potentials of the cells used cannot be eliminated.

Ion-Selective Electrode

Definition: Electrodes that exhibit a selective and sensitive response to certain ions in the solution are known as ion-selective electrode.

The glass-electrode is an ion-selective electrode which is sensitive to H_3O^+. By carefully controlling the composition of glass, the glass membrane shows its sensitiveness to monovalent ions such as sodium and potassium. The glass surface acts as ion exchanger and the certain ions can be held strongly at the surface-binding sites depending upon the composition of glass.

- Mobility of ions through the glass can be controlled by the modifications in the glass lattice structure.

- With these membrane electrodes, complete selectivity cannot be achieved because the glass response cannot be made completely independent of Hydrogen and other ions in the solution.

- The sensing barriers of the ion-selective electrode operates through the selective exchange of ions between two solutions on either side of the barrier.

- Potentials arising owing to the concentration differences between the solutions as well as from the resistance of the barriers.

- Salt crystals, liquids and enzymes as well as glass membranes are use either as single or sometimes incorporated into the matrix such as plastic to form a sensing barrier.

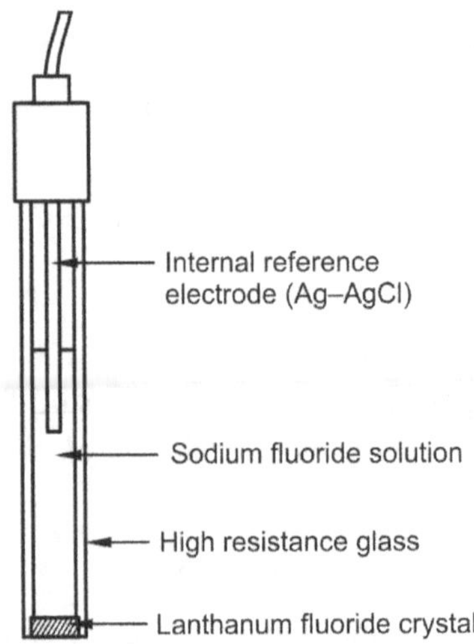

Fig. 8.8 Flouride Selective electrode.

An example of salt type barrier is fluoride-sensitive electrode which uses a fluoride salt of one of the lanthanum elements as an insoluble membrane.

Example: A crystal containing lanthanum fluoride or praseodymium or Europium fluoride (PrF_3 (or) EuF_3) can be sealed into the end of electrode. An inner filling solution of a known activity α of NaF is used with an internal reference electrode such as silver-silver chloride electrode.

The cell is represented as:

Internal reference NaF(α) | LaF3 crystal | External test solution (F $^-$ Electrode unknown concentration)

The potential difference across the LaF_3 crystal is due to the conductance of F ions, unless the ions are present in applicable concentration in the test solution. The electrode is practically free from other ions and can be considered selective for fluoride ion.

Structure of Valinomycin

For biologic samples, the fluoride concentration as low as 10^{-6} M can be determined quickly and this can be done only by a dilution or solubilisation step after the calibration. Accuracy of the method is $\pm 10\%$ for solution and the pH is in between 4 and 8 for this solution. At high pH values interference of Hydroxide ion occurs and at low pH values fluoride complexes and hydrofluoric acid.

Membrane carriers can be made from with the use of two substances.

1. Electrically neutral substances

2. Water-insoluble sensors.

The compound is incorporated into a plastic matrix such as polyvinylchloride (PVC) matrix.

The membrane sensor is made by mixing the sensor with a suitable solvent followed by addition of PVC and then mixing and finally removing the solvent. This membrane can be used directly as a barrier. One of the most selective widely used antibiotic is valinomycin.

This valinomycin has a 36-membered using structure and it acts as a selective complexing agent for potassium ions.

Mechanism: It involves cation-exchange across the antibiotic membrane to produce a potential between solution on either side.

Selectivity: It shows a selectivity of 4000:1 for k^+ over Na^+ ions and a selectivity of 20,000:1 for k^+ over H^+ ions.

It has linear potential response over the region from about 10^{-5} to 10^{-1}M for k^+ ions.

The electrode is represented as:

Internal reference electrode	KCl (known concentration)	External test solution (k^+ unknown concentration)

Charged ion exchangers, such as phosphate diesters can also be used as sensors. The compound can be dissolved in a solution which is in contact with a porous membrane that acts as a barrier and a junction to the test solution. An enzyme can be incorporated into the polyacrylonitrile plastic film which acts as a part of sensing barrier.

e.g.: An enzyme, urease which converts the urea into Ammonium ions

$$urea + H_2O \xrightarrow{HCO_3^-} HCO_3 + NH_4^+$$

This enzyme is immobile in the plastic matrix which is attached to a glass membrane electrode.

The glass membrane is sensitive to Ammonium ions. These Ammonium ions migrate through the plastic membrane to the glass surface. This can be easily be detected by change in potential. This electrode can detect urea in solution whose concentration within the range 10^{-4} to 10^{-2} M.

This ion-selective electrode produces a potential which is directly proportional to the logarithm of the activity of the ion.

The equation is

$$E_{cell} = E_{constant} + \frac{0.0592}{n} \log (\alpha) \quad\quad ..... (8.102)$$

where α is the activity of the ion.

Ionic strength of the standards is usually adjusted by treating each solution with an appropriate buffer of high molarity which eliminates the errors.

The EMF of a cell along with ion-selective electrode is called expanded pH-scale meter. The advantage is it can be used with a high-resistance input and allows 100-millivolt portion and the accurate EMF values are obtained.

Ion-selective electrodes are used to determine the dissolution rate of tablets, especially alkali containing tablets.

The release of sodium Phenobarbital through a dialyzing membrane can be monitored by using the dialyzed solution with sodium-selective electrode.

Redox potentials

An ion is said to be oxidized if it denotes electron to another ion and this ion is further reduced by accepting the denoted electrons.

e.g: Ferrous ion loses an electron and get converted to ferric ion. This is mainly due to oxidation.

e.g: $$Fe^{2+} + e^- \rightleftharpoons Fe^{3+} \quad\quad ..... (8.103)$$

This ferric ion gains an electron and gets converted to ferrous ion:

e.g: $$Fe^{3+} + e^- \rightleftharpoons Fe^{2+} \quad\quad ..... (8.104)$$

This can be expressed in the form of the following equation,

$$Red \rightleftharpoons ox + ne \quad\quad ..... (8.105)$$

where

Red = Reduced state (Reductant)

ox = Oxidized state (Oxidant)

ne = no. of electrons involved in the reaction.

Oxidation-Reduction (Redox) systems can be studied in a similar manner to pH system by using an inert indicator electrode (Eg: platinum) along with reference electrode (*e.g*: calomel electrode). The EMF depends upon the relative concentrations of oxidant and reductant. This potential is represented as En which is given by the Nernst equation:

$$E_n = E^0 + \frac{0.0592}{n} \log \frac{[ox]}{[Red]} \qquad \text{at 25 °C} \qquad \qquad ..... (8.106)$$

Where $\quad$ n = no. of electrons transferred per ion

$\qquad E^0$ = standard oxidation-reduction potential.

when the concentrations of oxidant and reductant are equal i.e., oxidant = Reductant

Substituting this in the above Nernst equation, it becomes,

$$E_n = E^0 + \frac{0.0592}{n} \log \frac{[ox]}{[ox]}$$

$$E_n = E^0 + \frac{0.0592}{n} \log (1) \qquad \qquad (\log 1 = 0)$$

$$E_n = E^0 + (0)$$

$$E_n = E^0$$

The potential E_n can be determined with the use of potentiometer in order to measure the potential difference between the indicator electrode (whose potential is E_h) and the reference electrode (E_{ref}) according to the following relationship

$$E_{cell} = E_{ref} - E_n \qquad \qquad ..... (8.107)$$

The E^0 of a redox system is a characteristic constant and it is a measure of its oxidizing or reducing tendency.

The Higher the E^0 value, the greater is the oxidizing ability of the system and conversely.

An example for the Redox potential is Quinhydrone electrode which was discussed under electrometric determination of pH .

During this determination in order to measure the accurate E_h use of certain dyes takes place. These dyes change their colour due to their change in the oxidation state.

e.g.: Methylene blue changes from colourless to deep blue at pH = 7 as e_n varies from 0.040 to – 0.062.

Redox indicators are used effectively to determine the equivalence point in Redox filtrations.

Determination of EMF of Sparingly Soluble Salts

The EMF of the sparingly soluble salts at 25 ^{0}C is calculated by using the equation

$$E = \frac{0.0591}{n} \log \frac{c_2}{c_1} \qquad \text{..... (8.108)}$$

In the case of sparingly soluble salt, the salt can be supposed to be completely ionized even in saturated solution.

The ionic concentration is proportional to the solubility of the salt.

e.g: The EMF of the cell

$$\text{Ag} \mid \text{Ag} \mid \text{in 0.045M KI} \parallel \text{0.045m AgNO}_3 \mid \text{Ag in 0.788 at 25°C}$$

Calculate:

1. the solubility product of AgI

2. solubility of Ag in water at 25 ^{0}C.

Sol: At 25 ^{0}C, the concentration of Ag^+ in the cathodic half-cell is 0.045M and the concentration of I oin anodic half-cell is 0.045M KI

(i) Let the concentration of AgI be c_1

$$E = \frac{0.0591}{1} \log \frac{0.045}{c_1}$$

$$0.788 = \frac{0.0591}{1} \log \frac{0.045}{c_1}$$

$$\log \frac{0.045}{c_1} = \frac{0.788}{0.0591} = 13.33$$

$$\frac{0.045}{c_1} = 2.138 \times 10^{13}$$

$$C_1 = \frac{0.045}{2.138 \times 10^{13}} = 2.105 \times 10^{-15}$$

(ii) The solubility of AgI $= \sqrt{k_{sp}}$

$$= \sqrt{9.472 \times 10^{-17}}$$
$$= 9.732 \times 10^{-9} \text{ g mol litre}^{-1}$$
$$= 9.732 \times 10^{-9} \times 143.5 \text{ g litre}^{-1}$$
$$= 1.396 \times 10^{-6} \text{ g litre}^{-1}$$

Determination of Valence

The EMF, E, of a concentration cell is

$$E = \frac{0.059}{n} \log_{10} \frac{c_2}{c_1}$$

e.g.: The following cell is constructed

$$Hg|\ 0.05\ N\ Hg_2\ (NO_3)_2\ \|\ 0.5N\ Hg_2\ (NO_3)_2\ |\ Hg$$

and its emf is found to be 0.029 v.

Sol: Let c_1 be the concentration of mercury ion in 0.05N Hg_2 $(NO_3)_2$ solution in the left half-cell and c_2 be the concentration of mercurous ion 0.5N Hg $(NO_3)_2$ solution in the right half-cell.

Substituting these values in above formulae:

$$0.029 = \frac{0.0591}{n} \log \frac{0.5}{0.05}$$

$$= \frac{0.0591}{n} \log 10 = \frac{0.0591}{n}$$

$$n = \frac{0.0591}{0.029}$$

$$n = 2.$$

8.6 Questions

1. With a neat labelled diagram explain the construction and working of Daniel cell.

2. What is the role of the salt bridge and how does it prevent accumulation of charges at the electrodes.

3. Define a cell and mention different types of electrodes and discuss the calomel Electrode.

CHAPTER 9

VISCOSITY

9.1 Introduction

Rheology is a Greek word where Rheo means flow and logos means science. It is the study of flow or deformation under stress. Viscosity in general terms is the resistance to flow. Coefficient of viscosity often called viscosity is the proportionality constant between the Rate of shear and shearing stress and therefore viscosity can be defined as "the ratio between the shearing stress and rate of shear".

When a force is applied on a fluid, it flows. When this force is removed the fluid either gas or liquid does not attain its original state. This signifies that in fluids irreversible deformation occurs.

A fluid can be considered as the summation of infinitesimally thin layers and when a deformation force is applied shearing is seen between different layers and the layers and the wall of the container. The deformation is expressed as rate of shear and the force applied as shear stress and therefore the definition of viscosity:

"Shearing force can be defined as the force applied to produce a deformation of 1 cm^2 area in the liquid" Thus

$$\text{Shearing stress} = \frac{F}{A} \qquad \text{.....(9.1)}$$

$$S = \frac{F}{A}$$

where F = Applied force (tangentially);   A = Surface area

"Shearing strain or stress or rate of shear can be defined as the rate at which the velocity V changes with the distance × perpendicular to direction of flow."

$$\text{Shearing strain} = D = \frac{dv}{dx} \qquad \text{.....(9.2)}$$

where dv = change in velocity

dx = change in distance perpendicular to direction of flow

From the definition of viscosity

$$\eta = \frac{S}{D} \qquad \text{.....(9.3)}$$

From eq. 9.1 and eq. 9.2 viscosity (η) becomes:

$$\eta = \frac{F}{A} \times \frac{dx}{dv} \qquad \text{.....(9.4)}$$

From eq. 9.4 units of viscosity can be evaluated as:

$$\text{C.G.S units :} \quad \frac{\text{dynes} \times \text{sec}}{\text{cm}^2} \quad \text{or} \quad \frac{g}{\text{cm} \times \text{sec}}$$

But viscosity is expressed as poise as a tribute to the works of poiseullie

1 centi poise = 0.01 poise

The accurate definition of viscosity can be given as "the shearing force required to produce a velocity of 1 cm/sec between two parallel plates of liquid each of 1 cm^2 in area and separated by a distance of 1cm."

Viscosity can also be expressed in:

Pascal second or millipascal second

1 millipascal second = 1 centi poise

$$1 \text{ pascal} = \frac{\text{Newton}}{\text{m}^2}$$

$$1 \text{ pascal} = \frac{\text{kilogram} \times \text{m}}{\text{sec}^2} \times \frac{1}{\text{m}^2}$$

$$= \frac{\text{kilogram}}{\text{sec}^2 \times \text{m}}$$

$$1 \text{ pascal second} = \frac{\text{kilogram}}{\text{sec} \times \text{m}}$$

$$= \text{Kg sec}^{-1} \text{ m}^{-1}$$

$$1 \text{ millipascal second} = \text{gm cm}^{-1} \text{ sec}^{-1}$$

Under general condition viscosity can be explained by considering the liquid existing between two large parallel plates. It is said that liquid exists as infinitesimally thin layers like deck of cards parallel to each other and finally parallel to the very large parallel plates. When the top plate is pushed or pulled the layers of liquid immediately below it moves in the same direction with the same velocity. If this layers is the 1st layers then the layer below it that is the second layer moves in the same direction but with the velocity less than the 1st layer. The 3rd layer will move with comparatively less velocity than the 2nd layer. This process continuous. The movement is because of drag force and friction between the layers.

Finally the bottom layers adhering to the stationary plate remains stationary with 'O' velocity. Thus the velocity of liquid layers is said to increase in the direction $\times$ perpendicular to the direction of movement of upper plane.

9.2 Applications of viscosity in pharmacy

The principles of viscosity can be applied in the field of pharmacy in the following ways:

1. In levigation and mixing of ointments on slabes
2. During preparation of suspensions and emulsions using molar and pestle.
3. During use of roller mills for compacting powders and processing ointments.
4. During flow of emulsions through colloidal mills and pumps.
5. In studying the mechanical properties of glass, plastic containers and rubber, polymeric closures.
6. In study of fluidity of injectables and intravenousy infused solutions.
7. In study of strength of sutures and ligatures.
8. Ease of pourability from a bottle, squeezing from a tube or other deformable containers.
9. Maintaining product shape in jars and after extrusion.
10. During rubbing the product onto the skin.

11. Rheology is also used as computational, Bio Rheology, clinical Hemorphology in microcirculation, absorptive rates of drugs and studying rheological properties of cerebrospinal fluid is much more important.

9.3 Flow of Liquids and Newtonian Fluids

The flow of liquids is best understood by knowing the works of Reynolds. He considered a straight transparent tube and introduced fluid (water) into it under the influence of flow. He maintained constant head of water.

At the centre of the inlet of the tube he introduced a fine stream of dye at low rates of flow. An undisturbed coherent thread was formed by the dye in the centre of the tube. This type of flow was then named as laminar flow. The liquid was considered to flow as series of concentric circles in laminar flow.

When the flow speed was increased to a critical velocity then the dye thread began to waver and thin broke up although mixing did not occur. This type of flow was called transitional flow.

When the flow velocity was further increased a high amount of dye instantaneously mixed with the fluid and irregular motion was imposed. Such flow was described as turbulent flow.

Reynolds work has proved that flow depends on four factors namely:

> diameter of pipe (d)
>
> viscosity of fluid (η)
>
> density of fluid (ρ) and
>
> velocity of fluid (v)

These factors were combined as follows to get Reynolds number

$$R_e = \frac{\rho v d}{\eta} \qquad \qquad .....(9.5)$$

Reynolds number is a dimensionless figure. When Reynolds number is below 2000 the flow is streamline and when Reynolds number is above 4000 the flow is turbulent.

9.4 Temperature Dependence of Viscosity

The aspect of dependence of temperature on viscosity is dealt in both gases and liquids.

In case of gases as the temperature increases viscosity of a gas increases. This is because when temperature of a gas is increased. The molecules of the gas collide to the space available and cause the increase in instantaneous density and therefore on increase in viscosity is observed.

Where as in case of liquids when temperature increases, the molecules move apart even vapourise and get lost from the liquid state. This leads to decrease in instantaneous density and thereby a decrease in viscosity. For liquids this relationship between viscosity and temperature is put forward as follows:

$$\eta = Ae^{E_vRT} \qquad \qquad .....(9.6)$$

$$ln\,\eta = \frac{E_v}{RT} + l\,n\,A \qquad \qquad .....(9.7)$$

where $\quad$ E_v = activation energy

$\qquad$ A = constant depending on molecular weight of liquid

$\qquad$ R = universal gas constant

$\qquad$ T = absolute temperature

The viscosity of many liquids decrease by about 2% with the rise of 1 °C in the temperature.

9.5 Types of viscosities

9.5.1 Kinematic Viscosity

It is the ratio between the Newtonian viscosity and density.

Practically viscosity is expressed as this type of kinematic viscosity.

$$\text{Kinematic viscosity (v)} = \frac{\eta}{\rho} \qquad \qquad .....(9.8)$$

where $\quad$ η = Newtonian viscosity

$\qquad$ ρ = density

Units of kinematic viscosity are strokes and centistrokes. Newtonian viscosity is nothing but dynamic viscosity.

9.5.2 Relative Viscosity:

Relative viscosity is the ratio between viscosity of the solution to viscosity of solvent alone

$$\text{Relative viscosity } (\eta_r) = \frac{\eta}{\eta_o} \qquad \qquad .....(9.9)$$

$\qquad$ η = viscosity of solution

$\qquad$ η_o = viscosity of solvent

9.5.3 Specific Viscosity

Specific viscosity can be defined as the ratio between the difference in the viscosity of solution and viscosity of solvent and that of viscosity of the solvent

$$\text{Specific viscosity } (\eta_s) = \left(\frac{\eta - \eta_o}{\eta_o} \right) \qquad \qquad .....(9.10)$$

$$\eta_s = \frac{\eta}{\eta_o} - 1$$

where η = viscosity of the solution

η_o = viscosity of the solvent

9.6 Determination of Viscosity

Measuring of viscosity includes following three basic and principle methods:

1. Based on rate of flow of liquid through an orfice or a duct of simple geometry such as "Capillary viscometer."

2. Based on resistance of rotating element which remains in contact with liquid even immersed in liquid such as "concentric cylinder viscometer."

3. Based on velocity of an object falling or rolling through the liquid which lies under effect of gravity such as "falling or rolling sphere viscometer."

9.6.1 Capillary Viscometer

A capillary viscometer can be used to determine viscosity to Newtonian fluids and fluids showing streamlined flow. The capillary viscometers most commonly used are:

Canon Fenske viscometer; Uubbelohde viscometer and Ostwald's viscometer.

In capillary viscometers, duct is a cylindrical capillary and the flow causing liquids to flow is its own weight.

9.6.2 Ostwald's Viscometer

This is a standard instrument even described in pharmacopocias was and meets the specifications of international standards organisation. An appropriate bore size must be selected such that flow time is approximately 200 seconds. Wider bore viscometers are used for high viscous fluids.

Construction of Ostwalds Viscometer: Ostwald's viscometer consists of a bent U shaped tube with two openings or bores. Each bore is said to be held by a tube and both the tubes meet at U bend. One tube contains bulb at a lower 3/4th end, other tube contains bulb at an upper 3/4th end. A capillary tube arises and travels little way from the bulb at the upper end. This capillary actually increases the time of flow of fluid from the bulb. Marks 'A' and 'B' are present above and below the bulb at the higher $3/4^{th}$ end and a mark G is present at the bulb at lower $3/4^{th}$ end of other tube.

Principle: The rate of flow of liquid through the tubes was given by poiseullie's equation as follows:

$$\frac{V}{t} = \frac{\pi P r^4}{8 \eta l} \qquad .....(9.11)$$

where   V = volume of liquid flowing in time t

P = pressure difference across the ends of the tube

r and *l* are radius and length of the tube

η = coefficient of viscosity

From the eq.9.11, if we want to compare the viscosities of two liquids r and *l* can be kept constant by using the same viscometer

Then we can write

$$\frac{V}{t} \propto \frac{P}{\eta} \qquad .....(9.12)$$

Pressure depends on hydrostatic head of the liquids which in turn depends on difference in heights of liquids in two arms of the V tube viscometer. If height difference is h and density is ρ and g = acceleration due to gravity.

$$\text{hydrostatic pressure (P)} = h\rho g \qquad .....(9.13)$$

on substituting eq. 9.13 in eq. 9.12

$$\frac{V}{t} \propto \frac{h\rho\rho}{\eta} \qquad .....(9.14)$$

V and h are also constant for a given viscometer along with r and *l*, by taking same amount of liquid each time.

Thus,

$$\frac{1}{t} \propto \frac{\rho}{\eta} \qquad .....(9.15)$$

But $\dfrac{\eta}{\rho}$ is called kinematic viscosity (V)

Thus $\dfrac{\eta}{\rho} \propto t$ and $V \propto t$ $\qquad .....(9.16)$

$$V = ct \qquad .....(9.17)$$

Thus

$$\frac{t_1}{t_2} = \frac{V_1}{V_2}$$

$$\frac{t_1}{t_2} = \frac{\eta_1}{\eta_2} \frac{P_2}{P_1}$$

$$\frac{\eta_1}{\eta_2} = \frac{P_1}{P_2} \frac{t_1}{t_2} \qquad\qquad .....(9.18)$$

where the constant in eq. 9.17 depends on V, h, r and *l*.

Experimental Corrections and Precautions

During working with capillary viscometer a viscometer must be selected in such a way that:

1. Streamline flow occurs in the capillary tube during experimentation.
2. Long unnecessary flow times are avoided
3. Capillary tube operates at 'single point' that means it operates at single shear rate.

9.7 Questions

1. Define viscosity and mention its types.
2. How do you determine the viscosity of a liquid.
3. Write the principle, derivation and working of Ostwald viscometer. Explain the method of determination of viscosity of a liquid by Ostwald viscometer with diagram.

CHAPTER 10

PHOTOCHEMISTRY

10.1 Introduction

The study of reactions caused by absorption of sunlight in the visible and UV light is called photochemistry. Visible light has a wavelength of (400-800 nm), UV light has a wavelength of (200-400 nm). Occurrence of any chemical reactions depends upon the activation of reactants. Reacting molecules acquire this activation energy by increasing their kinetic energy contrary to this, in case of photochemical reactions reaction molecules acquire the activation energy by the absorption of light energy (radiation).

Absorption Phenomenon of Electromagnetic Reaction and Consequences of Light Absorption

Light is said to possess small pockets of energy called quanta. In the atomic structure all the electrons in the ground state are paired. Each member of pair possesses an opposite spin in accordance with pauli's principle. The electrons present in the ground state absorbs quanta when light falls on them. This quantum energy source cause excitation of the electron to a higher transition state also called electronically excited state from its ground level. The promoted electron now has the same spin as its former partner on the opposite spin.

The electronically excited state has higher energy than the ground state. In ground state electrons are assigned to orbital labelled

sigma (σ).

Pi (π)

Non bonding (n) – lone pair

Antibonding (π^*) – with no paired electrons

Electronic transition may occur in these orbital.

$n \rightarrow \pi^*$ represents the excitation of an electron from a non bonding orbital n to antibonding orbital π^*.

Similarly $\pi \rightarrow \pi^*$ transition may occur.

- A molecule in which all the electrons are in paired, condition is said to be in singlet state (S).

- A molecule in which 2 electrons are unpaired is said to be in a triplet state (T).

Singlet state is confirmed by the antiparallel spins of parallel electrons according to pauli's exclusion principle.

Excited State, Ground State and Energy Transitions

Light of any wavelength is associated with an energy value given by

$$E = h\nu \qquad\qquad\qquad .....(10.1)$$

where   E = energy

h = planks constant,

ν = frequency

Frequency: Frequency of light can be defined as the ratio between the velocity of light C and wavelength of light λ

$$\nu = \frac{C}{\lambda} \qquad\qquad\qquad .....(10.2)$$

As discussed earlier energy is quantised (consists of well defined packets called quanta (plural) quantum (singular). The energy quantity required to raise an electron from one level to a higher level in a given molecule is a fixed quantity. The light source with frequency corresponding to this fixed quantity only can cause the transition of electrons in the molecule. If a light is either too high or too low frequency passes through the molecule unchanged. If the light of correct frequency is passed, the energy will be used by the molecules and hence light that leaves the molecules will be of diminished intensity. The photoexcitation process is rapid. It is even faster than a molecular vibration. In most cases triplet state has less energy compared to the singlet state.

10.2 Beer-lamberts Law

When a beam of light is passed through a transparent cell containing a solution of an absorbing substance a reduction in the intensity of light may be observed. This is due to:

1. Rejections of the light at the inner and outer surfaces of the cell.

2. Scattering by the particles in the solution.

3. Absorption of light by the molecules in the solution

The reflections of the light at the inner and outer surface of the cell can be compensated by a reference cell containing solvent only.

The scattering by the particles in the solution can be eliminated by filtration of the solution.

The intensity of light absorbed can be given by:

$$I_{absorbed} = I_o - I_T \qquad\qquad .....(10.3)$$

where I_o is the original intensity

I_T is the reduced intensity (transmitted from the cell)

Transmittance (T) is the ratio between I_T / I_o

$$T = \frac{I_T}{I_o} \qquad\qquad .....(10.4)$$

Percentage transmission is given

$$\%T = \frac{100\, I_T}{I_o} \qquad\qquad .....(10.5)$$

Lambert investigated the relationship between I_T and I_o for various thicknesses of substances inside the cell.

He found that the rate of decrease in intensity of the light with the thickness, b, of the medium is proportional to the intensity of the incident light

$$-\frac{dI}{db} \propto I \qquad \text{(or)}$$

$$-\frac{dI}{db} = K^1 I \qquad \qquad .....(10.6)$$

where K^1 is a proportionality constant

On integrating and converting into common logarithm the eq. 10.6 becomes

$$\log \frac{I_o}{I_T} = \frac{K'b}{2.303} \qquad .....(10.7)$$

where 'I_T' is the intensity at thickness 'b'.

The quantity $\log \frac{I_o}{I_T}$ is called absorbance (A)

Absorbance (A) is equal to the reciprocal of common logarithm of transmittance

$$A = \log_{10} \frac{I_o}{I_T}$$

$$= \log_{10} \left(\frac{1}{T}\right)$$

$$= -\log T$$

$$= -2 \log (\%T) \qquad .....(10.8)$$

10.2.1 Lambert's Law

Lambert's law can be defined as the intensity of a beam of parallel monochromatic radiation decrease exponentially as it passes through a medium of homogeneous thickness. In a simplified manner is stated that the absorbance is proportional to the thickness of the solution.

Beer showed that a similar relationship exists between the absorbance and the concentration

$$\log \frac{I_o}{I_T} = \frac{K''C}{2.303} \qquad ......(10.9)$$

where K'' is the proportionality constant

C is the concentration

10.2.2 Beer's Law

Beer's law is defined as the intensity of a beam of parallel monochromatic radiation decreases exponentially with the number of absorbing molecules.

In a simplified manner it is stated that the absorbance is proportional to the concentration.

When Beer's law and Lambert's Law are combined it gives Beer's-lamberts law.

$$A = \log \frac{I_o}{I_T} = abc \qquad\qquad .....(10.10)$$

The proportionality constant $\dfrac{K'}{2.303}$ of Lambert's law and $\dfrac{K''}{2.303}$ of Beer's law are combined to give **a**

Quantum efficiency ϕ : The determination of quantum yield or quantum efficiency is a consequence of determination of photochemical mechanisms. The fraction of absorbed light that is used to produce a particular result is nothing but quantum yield. It might be expected that one molecule would react for each quantum absorbed. This is called law of photochemical equivalence but is rarely observed in practice. The reason for this has been explained as follows:

Photochemical reactions generally consist of two processes. The first is the primary process in which the light has been absorbed to produce the excited molecule. If energy is high enough, dissociation occurs to give free radicals. This dissociation often involves fission of Carbon-Carbon single bonds, when a quantum of $\lambda = 300$ nm and $\Delta E = {\sim}398$ KJ/mol will bring about homolytic fission. This primary process is said to obey the law of photochemical equivalence and it later followed by secondary process. In the secondary process, the products of primary process undergo further reactions. Thus the total quantum yield or quantum efficiency of the process can be defined as

$$\text{Quantum yield} = \frac{Number \text{ of molecules reacting or produced}}{Number\ of\ quanta\ absorbed} \qquad .....(10.11)$$

The total quantum yield can also be called as product quantum yield.

Quantum yield oρ θυαντυμ εφφιχιενχψ ισ δεσιγνατεδ βψ ϕ. If we consider a product (P) that is formed from a photochemical reaction of an initially exited molecule A, ϕ can be written as

$$\phi = \frac{\text{Number of molecules of P formed}}{\text{Number of quanta absorbed by A}} \qquad .....(10.12)$$

Product quantum yields are much easier to measure. The number of quanta absorbed can be determined by an instrument called actinometer.

ϕ values varies from 10^{-2} to 10^4 and even more

ϕ value is rarely unity in practice

Secondary photochemical processes are of various types like substitution, addition, dimerisation, elimination, rearrangement etc.

INDEX

www.ingramcontent.com/pod-product-compliance
Lightning Source LLC
LaVergne TN
LVHW080049210726
843507LV00017B/707